The Big Book of

HAMILTON BEACH

Air Fryer

A COLLECTION OF 250 AIR FRYER RECIPES TO MANAGE YOUR HEALTH WITH STEP BY STEP INSTRUCTIONS

TIMOTHY DAVIDSON

CONTENTS

INTRODUCTION

Getting to Know the Hamilton Beach Air Fryer

Deep-frying your food may taste amazing, but it's certainly not beneficial for your health. Air fryers perform convective heat transfer, or convection: A heating element heats the surrounding air and then an internal fan rapidly circulates that heated air. Because the heated air is circulated, it makes contact with every bit of surface area on the food, crisping your food and creating a nice crust without the use of excessive oil and grease. In an air fryer, food typically sits in a perforated basket or on a wire rack inside the air fryer, which also facilitates contact between heated air and every surface of the food.

Seeing the Benefits of the Hamilton Beach Air Fryer

Healthier Cooking

Air fryers are a great option if you're looking for a healthy alternative to typically fatty foods. With an air fryer, you can cook all your favorite fried dishes without the unhealthy amount of oil present in their deep-fried versions. Air fryers are specifically designed to cook with less oil, producing food with up to 80% less fat than traditional fryers. You can cook without any oil at all, or you can toss your food in a small amount of oil before cooking for an extra crunch.

Quick Meals

Since they're smaller than an oven and circulate air more rapidly, air fryers cook food faster than other appliances. Air fryers can achieve high temperatures within minutes (or seconds), a process that usually takes at least 10 minutes with a traditional oven. An air fryer is a great option for you if you don't have a lot of time to cook meals. However, keep in mind that most air fryers can only cook so fast because of their small size, so if you have a large family, it may be hard for you to cook for everyone at once.

Adaptability

Air fryers are known for their extreme versatility. When we say they can cook almost anything, we mean it. You can cook fresh foods as well as frozen foods and even reheat leftovers. Remember, if you're looking for a frying effect, breaded foods do better than battered foods. Look for different accessories and attachments, such as additional fry baskets, baking racks, and cooking pans, to increase your air fryer's functionality even more!

Easy Cleanup

Cleanup – the dreaded process at the end of cooking. Air fryers make cleaning simpler at the end of meals. Most of their internal components are removable for easy cleaning. For added convenience, many are even dishwasher-safe. Easy cleanup can cut down on the amount of time you spend in the kitchen and encourage you to cook more often.

Tips and Tricks on How to Use the Hamilton Beach Air Fryer

Don't be intimated by the air fryer! Once you get the hang of it, you'll never know how you lived without it before. Try these tips to cook with your air fryer like a pro:

(1) Always Preheat Before Cooking – Think of your air fryer like a little oven. If yours doesn't have a preheat feature, allow it to warm up for 3-5 minutes before you begin cooking.

(2) Spray the Basket – Even if your recipe doesn't call for oil, be sure to spray the basket's bottom for best results! You can use cooking spray, butter, or grease it with a little olive oil.

(3) Don't Overfill the Basket – Cook in batches if you need to! It's important not to let your food overlap. If you try to squeeze too much in, you may end up with a soggy, undercooked mess. Easy does it!

(4) Flip or Shake Foods You Want Crispy – If you're cooking french fries or chicken wings, flip them halfway through or remove the basket and shake. This helps them crisp evenly.

(5) Invest in Baking Pans & Accessories – These air fryer accessories will make life so much easier and cleaning a breeze!

(6) Have Fun & Experiment – We think this tip is the most important! Once you get the hang of cooking with your air fryer, have some fun with it. Branch out and try new things! You'll get used to the cooking times, breading methods, and more, so use your knowledge to create new recipes.

Hints on Cleaning the Hamilton Beach Air Fryer

Cleaning and preserving are the most important factors to decide the durability of an appliance. The best time to clean an air fryer is immediately after use, which will ensure that food particles do not stick to the sides and become hard to remove. However, do not rush and let the machine cool down about 30 minutes before cleaning. Air fryers usually come with an instruction manual; hence, you can also refer to this manual to see how best you can care for your new device to extend the useful lifespan saving you money in the long term.

◆ Clean the frying basket

1) The bottom frying basket is where lots of grease and gunk falls, so cleaning it properly to prevent grease build-up and bacteria growth that could foul the foods and make you sick. You can proceed to clean the basket according to the following instructions:

2) Make sure that the device is unplugged from the power source and wait until it's cool to start cleaning. You can remove the air fryer basket and either set it in the sink or on the counter. This will help it cool down even faster.

3) Use a damp cloth to wipe down the exterior. Wipe away the soap with a clean damp cloth. And repeat this step for the interior.

4) Remove the basket and tray from the main unit, then use a bit of dish soap with warm water to wash them with a soft sponge or cloth—no abrasives.

5) If food is stuck on these components, you should soak them in hot soapy water for at least 10 minutes before scrubbing with a non-abrasive sponge.

6) Don't forget to dry it completely before you put it back in the air fryer!

7) It's a good idea to clean the frying basket after each use to ensure to remove all old foods and grease causes to smell and effects to the taste of food.

◆ Clean the Crumb Basket

1) Take the crumb basket out and throw away any loose pieces of food leftover in it. Wipe it out with a damp cloth.

2) Make sure you clean all the crevices and both the outside and inside of the basket. It might help to use a dish brush or toothbrush to clean all the slats.

3) Dry it completely. Make sure it completely dry before replacing them in the air fryer.

Note:

➢ The crumb basket has a non-stick coating on it, so please don't use abrasive brushes (like steel wool) on it or any abrasive cleaners that might erode this coating. This is why we do not recommend using a dishwasher. They operate at high heat which erodes the surface of the nonstick cookware. It can lead to flaking which can be toxic.

➢ We are also against using any strong detergents or things that aren't designed to clean. Often, these can have the opposite effect and actually cause damage instead of cleaning.

Bread And Breakfast

Baked Eggs

Servings: 4
Cooking Time: 6 Minutes
Ingredients:
- 4 large eggs
- ⅛ teaspoon black pepper
- ⅛ teaspoon salt

Directions:
1. Preheat the air fryer to 330°F. Place 4 silicone muffin liners into the air fryer basket.
2. Crack 1 egg at a time into each silicone muffin liner. Sprinkle with black pepper and salt.
3. Bake for 6 minutes. Remove and let cool 2 minutes prior to serving.

Soft Pretzels

Servings: 12
Cooking Time: 6 Minutes
Ingredients:
- 2 teaspoons yeast
- 1 cup water, warm
- 1 teaspoon sugar
- 1 teaspoon salt
- 2½ cups all-purpose flour
- 2 tablespoons butter, melted
- 1 cup boiling water
- 1 tablespoon baking soda
- coarse sea salt
- melted butter

Directions:
1. Combine the yeast and water in a small bowl. Combine the sugar, salt and flour in the bowl of a stand mixer. With the mixer running and using the dough hook, drizzle in the yeast mixture and melted butter and knead dough until smooth and elastic – about 10 minutes. Shape into a ball and let the dough rise for 1 hour.
2. Punch the dough down to release any air and decide what size pretzels you want to make.
3. a. To make large pretzels, divide the dough into 12 portions.
4. b. To make medium sized pretzels, divide the dough into 24 portions.
5. c. To make mini pretzel knots, divide the dough into 48 portions.
6. Roll each portion into a skinny rope using both hands on the counter and rolling from the center to the ends of the rope. Spin the rope into a pretzel shape (or tie the rope into a knot) and place the tied pretzels on a parchment lined baking sheet.
7. Preheat the air fryer to 350°F.
8. Combine the boiling water and baking soda in a shallow bowl and whisk to dissolve (this mixture will bubble, but it will settle down). Let the water cool so that you can put your hands in it. Working in batches, dip the pretzels (top side down) into the baking soda-water mixture and let them soak for 30 seconds to a minute. (This step is what gives pretzels their texture and helps them to brown faster.) Then, remove the pretzels carefully and return them (top side up) to the baking sheet. Sprinkle the coarse salt on the top.
9. Air-fry in batches for 3 minutes per side. When the pretzels are finished, brush them generously with the melted butter and enjoy them warm with some spicy mustard.

Hashbrown Potatoes Lyonnaise

Servings: 4
Cooking Time: 33 Minutes
Ingredients:
- 1 Vidalia (or other sweet) onion, sliced
- 1 teaspoon butter, melted
- 1 teaspoon brown sugar
- 2 large russet potatoes (about 1 pound), sliced ½-inch thick
- 1 tablespoon vegetable oil
- salt and freshly ground black pepper

Directions:
1. Preheat the air fryer to 370°F.
2. Toss the sliced onions, melted butter and brown sugar together in the air fryer basket. Air-fry for 8 minutes, shaking the basket occasionally to help the onions cook evenly.
3. While the onions are cooking, bring a 3-quart saucepan of salted water to a boil on the stovetop. Par-cook the potatoes in boiling water for 3 minutes. Drain the potatoes and pat them dry with a clean kitchen towel.
4. Add the potatoes to the onions in the air fryer basket and drizzle with vegetable oil. Toss to coat the potatoes with the oil and season with salt and freshly ground black pepper.
5. Increase the air fryer temperature to 400°F and air-fry for 22 minutes tossing the vegetables a few times during the cooking time to help the potatoes brown evenly. Season to taste again with salt and freshly ground black pepper and serve warm.

Pizza Dough

Servings: 3
Cooking Time: 10 Minutes
Ingredients:
- 4 cups bread flour, pizza ("00") flour or all-purpose flour
- 1 teaspoon active dry yeast
- 2 teaspoons sugar
- 2 teaspoons salt
- 1½ cups water
- 1 tablespoon olive oil

Directions:
1. Combine the flour, yeast, sugar and salt in the bowl of a stand mixer. Add the olive oil to the flour mixture and start to mix using the dough hook attachment. As you're mixing, add 1¼ cups of the water, mixing until the dough comes together. Continue to knead the dough with the dough hook for another 10 minutes, adding enough water to the dough to get it to the right consistency.
2. Transfer the dough to a floured counter and divide it into 3 equal portions. Roll each portion into a ball. Lightly coat each dough ball with oil and transfer to the refrigerator, covered with plastic wrap. You can place them all on a baking sheet, or place each dough ball into its own oiled zipper sealable plastic bag or container. (You can freeze the dough balls at this stage, removing as much air as possible from the oiled bag.) Keep in the refrigerator for at least one day, or as long as five days.
3. When you're ready to use the dough, remove your dough from the refrigerator at least 1 hour prior to baking and let it sit on the counter, covered gently with plastic wrap.

Garlic-cheese Biscuits

Servings: 8
Cooking Time: 8 Minutes
Ingredients:
- 1 cup self-rising flour
- 1 teaspoon garlic powder
- 2 tablespoons butter, diced
- 2 ounces sharp Cheddar cheese, grated
- ½ cup milk
- cooking spray

Directions:
1. Preheat air fryer to 330°F.
2. Combine flour and garlic in a medium bowl and stir together.
3. Using a pastry blender or knives, cut butter into dry ingredients.
4. Stir in cheese.
5. Add milk and stir until stiff dough forms.
6. If dough is too sticky to handle, stir in 1 or 2 more tablespoons of self-rising flour before shaping. Biscuits should be firm enough to hold their shape. Otherwise, they'll stick to the air fryer basket.
7. Divide dough into 8 portions and shape into 2-inch biscuits about ¾-inch thick.
8. Spray air fryer basket with nonstick cooking spray.
9. Place all 8 biscuits in basket and cook at 330°F for 8 minutes.

Egg Muffins

Servings: 4
Cooking Time: 11 Minutes
Ingredients:
- 4 eggs
- salt and pepper
- olive oil
- 4 English muffins, split
- 1 cup shredded Colby Jack cheese
- 4 slices ham or Canadian bacon

Directions:
1. Preheat air fryer to 390°F.
2. Beat together eggs and add salt and pepper to taste. Spray air fryer baking pan lightly with oil and add eggs. Cook for 2minutes, stir, and continue cooking for 4minutes, stirring every minute, until eggs are scrambled to your preference. Remove pan from air fryer.
3. Place bottom halves of English muffins in air fryer basket. Take half of the shredded cheese and divide it among the muffins. Top each with a slice of ham and one-quarter of the eggs. Sprinkle remaining cheese on top of the eggs. Use a fork to press the cheese into the egg a little so it doesn't slip off before it melts.
4. Cook at 360°F for 1 minute. Add English muffin tops and cook for 4minutes to heat through and toast the muffins.

Cinnamon Biscuit Rolls

Servings: 12
Cooking Time: 5 Minutes
Ingredients:
- Dough
- ¼ cup warm water (105–115°F)
- 1 teaspoon active dry yeast
- 1 tablespoon sugar
- ½ cup buttermilk, lukewarm
- 2 cups flour, plus more for dusting
- 1 teaspoon baking powder
- ½ teaspoon salt
- 3 tablespoons cold butter
- Filling
- 1 tablespoon butter, melted
- 1 teaspoon cinnamon

- 2 tablespoons sugar
- Icing
- ⅔ cup powdered sugar
- ¼ teaspoon vanilla
- 2–3 teaspoons milk

Directions:

1. Dissolve yeast and sugar in warm water. Add buttermilk, stir, and set aside.
2. In a large bowl, sift together flour, baking powder, and salt. Using knives or a pastry blender, cut in butter until mixture is well combined and crumbly.
3. Pour in buttermilk mixture and stir with fork until a ball of dough forms.
4. Knead dough on a lightly floured surface for 5minutes. Roll into an 8 x 11-inch rectangle.
5. For the filling, spread the melted butter over the dough.
6. In a small bowl, stir together the cinnamon and sugar, then sprinkle over dough.
7. Starting on a long side, roll up dough so that you have a roll about 11 inches long. Cut into 12 slices with a serrated knife and sawing motion so slices remain round.
8. Place rolls on a plate or cookie sheet about an inch apart and let rise for 30minutes.
9. For icing, mix the powdered sugar, vanilla, and milk. Stir and add additional milk until icing reaches a good spreading consistency.
10. Preheat air fryer to 360°F.
11. Place 6 cinnamon rolls in basket and cook 5 minutes or until top springs back when lightly touched. Repeat to cook remaining 6 rolls.
12. Spread icing over warm rolls and serve.

Western Frittata

Servings: 1
Cooking Time: 19 Minutes

Ingredients:

- ½ red or green bell pepper, cut into ½-inch chunks
- 1 teaspoon olive oil
- 3 eggs, beaten
- ¼ cup grated Cheddar cheese
- ¼ cup diced cooked ham
- salt and freshly ground black pepper, to taste
- 1 teaspoon butter
- 1 teaspoon chopped fresh parsley

Directions:

1. Preheat the air fryer to 400°F.
2. Toss the peppers with the olive oil and air-fry for 6 minutes, shaking the basket once or twice during the cooking process to redistribute the ingredients.
3. While the vegetables are cooking, beat the eggs well in a bowl, stir in the Cheddar cheese and ham, and season with salt and freshly ground black pepper. Add the air-fried peppers to this bowl when they have finished cooking.
4. Place a 6- or 7-inch non-stick metal cake pan into the air fryer basket with the butter using an aluminum sling to lower the pan into the basket. (Fold a piece of aluminum foil into a strip about 2-inches wide by 24-inches long.) Air-fry for 1 minute at 380°F to melt the butter. Remove the cake pan and rotate the pan to distribute the butter and grease the pan. Pour the egg mixture into the cake pan and return the pan to the air fryer, using the aluminum sling.
5. Air-fry at 380°F for 12 minutes, or until the frittata has puffed up and is lightly browned. Let the frittata sit in the air fryer for 5 minutes to cool to an edible temperature and set up. Remove the cake pan from the air fryer, sprinkle with parsley and serve immediately.

Parmesan Garlic Naan

Servings: 6
Cooking Time: 4 Minutes
Ingredients:
- 1 cup bread flour
- 1 teaspoon baking powder
- ⅛ teaspoon salt
- 1 teaspoon garlic powder
- 2 tablespoon shredded parmesan cheese
- 1 cup plain 2% fat Greek yogurt
- 1 tablespoon extra-virgin olive oil

Directions:
1. Preheat the air fryer to 400°F.
2. In a medium bowl, mix the flour, baking powder, salt, garlic powder, and cheese. Mix the yogurt into the flour, using your hands to combine if necessary.
3. On a flat surface covered with flour, divide the dough into 6 equal balls and roll each out into a 4-inch-diameter circle.
4. Lightly brush both sides of each naan with olive oil and place one naan at a time into the basket. Cook for 3 to 4 minutes (or until the bread begins to rise and brown on the outside). Remove and repeat for the remaining breads.
5. Serve warm.

Almond Cranberry Granola

Servings: 12
Cooking Time: 9 Minutes
Ingredients:
- 2 tablespoons sesame seeds
- ¼ cup chopped almonds
- ¼ cup sunflower seeds
- ½ cup unsweetened shredded coconut
- 2 tablespoons unsalted butter, melted or at least softened
- 2 tablespoons coconut oil
- ⅓ cup honey
- 2½ cups oats
- ¼ teaspoon sea salt
- ½ cup dried cranberries

Directions:
1. In a large mixing bowl, stir together the sesame seeds, almonds, sunflower seeds, coconut, butter, coconut oil, honey, oats, and salt.
2. Line the air fryer basket with parchment paper. Punch 8 to 10 holes into the parchment paper with a fork so air can circulate. Pour the granola mixture onto the parchment paper.
3. Air fry the granola at 350°F for 9 minutes, stirring every 3 minutes.
4. When cooking is complete, stir in the dried cranberries and allow the mixture to cool. Store in an airtight container up to 2 weeks or freeze for 6 months.

White Wheat Walnut Bread

Servings: 8
Cooking Time: 25 Minutes
Ingredients:
- 1 cup lukewarm water (105–115°F)
- 1 packet RapidRise yeast
- 1 tablespoon light brown sugar
- 2 cups whole-grain white wheat flour
- 1 egg, room temperature, beaten with a fork
- 2 teaspoons olive oil
- ½ teaspoon salt
- ½ cup chopped walnuts
- cooking spray

Directions:
1. In a small bowl, mix the water, yeast, and brown sugar.
2. Pour yeast mixture over flour and mix until smooth.

3. Add the egg, olive oil, and salt and beat with a wooden spoon for 2minutes.

4. Stir in chopped walnuts. You will have very thick batter rather than stiff bread dough.

5. Spray air fryer baking pan with cooking spray and pour in batter, smoothing the top.

6. Let batter rise for 15minutes.

7. Preheat air fryer to 360°F.

8. Cook bread for 25 minutes, until toothpick pushed into center comes out with crumbs clinging. Let bread rest for 10minutes before removing from pan.

Walnut Pancake

Servings: 4

Cooking Time: 20 Minutes

Ingredients:

- 3 tablespoons butter, divided into thirds
- 1 cup flour
- 1½ teaspoons baking powder
- ¼ teaspoon salt
- 2 tablespoons sugar
- ¾ cup milk
- 1 egg, beaten
- 1 teaspoon pure vanilla extract
- ½ cup walnuts, roughly chopped
- maple syrup or fresh sliced fruit, for serving

Directions:

1. Place 1 tablespoon of the butter in air fryer baking pan. Cook at 330°F for 3minutes to melt.

2. In a small dish or pan, melt the remaining 2 tablespoons of butter either in the microwave or on the stove.

3. In a medium bowl, stir together the flour, baking powder, salt, and sugar. Add milk, beaten egg, the 2 tablespoons of melted butter, and vanilla. Stir until combined but do not beat. Batter may be slightly lumpy.

4. Pour batter over the melted butter in air fryer baking pan. Sprinkle nuts evenly over top.

5. Cook for 20minutes or until toothpick inserted in center comes out clean. Turn air fryer off, close the machine, and let pancake rest for 2minutes.

6. Remove pancake from pan, slice, and serve with syrup or fresh fruit.

Country Gravy

Servings: 2

Cooking Time: 7 Minutes

Ingredients:

- ¼ pound pork sausage, casings removed
- 1 tablespoon butter
- 2 tablespoons flour
- 2 cups whole milk
- ½ teaspoon salt
- freshly ground black pepper
- 1 teaspoon fresh thyme leaves

Directions:

1. Preheat a saucepan over medium heat. Add and brown the sausage, crumbling it into small pieces as it cooks. Add the butter and flour, stirring well to combine. Continue to cook for 2 minutes, stirring constantly.

2. Slowly pour in the milk, whisking as you do, and bring the mixture to a boil to thicken. Season with salt and freshly ground black pepper, lower the heat and simmer until the sauce has thickened to your desired consistency – about 5 minutes. Stir in the fresh thyme, season to taste and serve hot.

Strawberry Toast

Servings: 4

Cooking Time: 8 Minutes

Ingredients:

- 4 slices bread, ½-inch thick
- butter-flavored cooking spray
- 1 cup sliced strawberries
- 1 teaspoon sugar

Directions:

1. Spray one side of each bread slice with butter-flavored cooking spray. Lay slices sprayed side down.
2. Divide the strawberries among the bread slices.
3. Sprinkle evenly with the sugar and place in the air fryer basket in a single layer.
4. Cook at 390°F for 8minutes. The bottom should look brown and crisp and the top should look glazed.

Sweet Potato-cinnamon Toast

Servings: 6

Cooking Time: 8 Minutes

Ingredients:

- 1 small sweet potato, cut into ⅜-inch slices
- oil for misting
- ground cinnamon

Directions:

1. Preheat air fryer to 390°F.
2. Spray both sides of sweet potato slices with oil. Sprinkle both sides with cinnamon to taste.
3. Place potato slices in air fryer basket in a single layer.
4. Cook for 4minutes, turn, and cook for 4 more minutes or until potato slices are barely fork tender.

Christmas Eggnog Bread

Servings: 6

Cooking Time: 18 Minutes

Ingredients:

- 1 cup flour, plus more for dusting
- ¼ cup sugar
- 1 teaspoon baking powder
- ¼ teaspoon salt
- ¼ teaspoon nutmeg
- ½ cup eggnog
- 1 egg yolk
- 1 tablespoon butter, plus 1 teaspoon, melted
- ¼ cup pecans
- ¼ cup chopped candied fruit (cherries, pineapple, or mixed fruits)
- cooking spray

Directions:

1. Preheat air fryer to 360°F.
2. In a medium bowl, stir together the flour, sugar, baking powder, salt, and nutmeg.
3. Add eggnog, egg yolk, and butter. Mix well but do not beat.
4. Stir in nuts and fruit.
5. Spray a 6 x 6-inch baking pan with cooking spray and dust with flour.
6. Spread batter into prepared pan and cook at 360°F for 18 minutes or until top is dark golden brown and bread starts to pull away from sides of pan.

Pepperoni Pizza Bread

Servings: 4

Cooking Time: 15 Minutes

Ingredients:

- 7-inch round bread boule
- 2 cups grated mozzarella cheese
- 1 tablespoon dried oregano
- 1 cup pizza sauce
- 1 cup mini pepperoni or pepperoni slices, cut in quarters
- Pizza sauce for dipping (optional)

Directions:

1. Make 7 to 8 deep slices across the bread boule, leaving 1 inch of bread uncut at the bottom of every slice before you reach the cutting board. The slices should go about three quarters of the way through the boule and be about 2 inches apart from each other. Turn the bread boule 90 degrees and make 7 to 8 similar slices perpendicular to the first slices to form squares in the bread. Again, make sure you don't cut all the way through the bread.

2. Combine the mozzarella cheese and oregano in a small bowl.

3. Fill the slices in the bread with pizza sauce by gently spreading the bread apart and spooning the sauce in between the squares of bread. Top the sauce with the mozzarella cheese mixture and then the pepperoni. Do your very best to get the cheese and pepperoni in between the slices, rather than on top of the bread. Keep spreading the bread apart and stuffing the ingredients in, but be careful not to tear the bottom of the bread.

4. Preheat the air fryer to 320°F.

5. Transfer the bread boule to the air fryer basket and air-fry for 15 minutes, making sure the top doesn't get too dark. (It will just be the cheese on top that gets dark, so if you've done a good job of tucking the cheese in between the slices, this shouldn't be an issue.)

6. Carefully remove the bread from the basket with a spatula. Transfer it to a serving platter with more sauce to dip into if desired. Serve with a lot of napkins so that people can just pull the bread apart with their hands and enjoy!

Southern Sweet Cornbread

Servings: 6

Cooking Time: 17 Minutes

Ingredients:

- cooking spray
- ½ cup white cornmeal
- ½ cup flour
- 2 teaspoons baking powder
- ½ teaspoon salt
- 4 teaspoons sugar
- 1 egg
- 2 tablespoons oil
- ½ cup milk

Directions:

1. Preheat air fryer to 360°F.

2. Spray air fryer baking pan with nonstick cooking spray.

3. In a medium bowl, stir together the cornmeal, flour, baking powder, salt, and sugar.

4. In a small bowl, beat together the egg, oil, and milk. Stir into dry ingredients until well combined.

5. Pour batter into prepared baking pan.

6. Cook at 360°F for 17 minutes or until toothpick inserted in center comes out clean or with crumbs clinging.

Crispy Bacon

Servings: 6

Cooking Time: 20 Minutes

Ingredients:

- 12 ounces bacon

Directions:

1. Preheat the air fryer to 350°F for 3 minutes.
2. Lay out the bacon in a single layer, slightly overlapping the strips of bacon.
3. Air fry for 10 minutes or until desired crispness.
4. Repeat until all the bacon has been cooked.

Banana Bread

Servings: 6

Cooking Time: 20 Minutes

Ingredients:

- cooking spray
- 1 cup white wheat flour
- ½ teaspoon baking powder
- ¼ teaspoon salt
- ¼ teaspoon baking soda
- 1 egg
- ½ cup mashed ripe banana
- ¼ cup plain yogurt
- ¼ cup pure maple syrup
- 2 tablespoons coconut oil
- ½ teaspoon pure vanilla extract

Directions:

1. Preheat air fryer to 330°F.
2. Lightly spray 6 x 6-inch baking dish with cooking spray.
3. In a medium bowl, mix together the flour, baking powder, salt, and soda.
4. In a separate bowl, beat the egg and add the mashed banana, yogurt, syrup, oil, and vanilla. Mix until well combined.
5. Pour liquid mixture into dry ingredients and stir gently to blend. Do not beat. Batter may be slightly lumpy.
6. Pour batter into baking dish and cook at 330°F for 20 minutes or until toothpick inserted in center of loaf comes out clean.

English Scones

Servings: 8

Cooking Time: 8 Minutes

Ingredients:

- 2 cups all-purpose flour
- 1 tablespoon baking powder
- ½ teaspoon salt
- 2 tablespoons sugar
- ¼ cup unsalted butter
- ⅔ cup plus 1 tablespoon whole milk, divided

Directions:

1. Preheat the air fryer to 380°F.
2. In a large bowl, whisk together the flour, baking powder, salt, and sugar. Using a pastry blender or your fingers, cut in the butter until pea-size crumbles appear. Make a well in the center and pour in ⅔ cup of the milk. Quickly mix the batter until a ball forms. Knead the dough 3 times.
3. Place the dough onto a floured surface and, using your hands or a rolling pin, flatten the dough until it's ¾ inch thick. Using a biscuit cutter or drinking glass, cut out 10 circles, reforming the dough and flattening as needed to use up the batter.
4. Brush the tops lightly with the remaining 1 tablespoon of milk.
5. Place the scones into the air fryer basket. Cook for 8 minutes or until golden brown and cooked in the center.

Blueberry Muffins

Servings: 8
Cooking Time: 14 Minutes

Ingredients:

- 1⅓ cups flour
- ½ cup sugar
- 2 teaspoons baking powder
- ¼ teaspoon salt
- ⅓ cup canola oil
- 1 egg
- ½ cup milk
- ⅔ cup blueberries, fresh or frozen and thawed
- 8 foil muffin cups including paper liners

Directions:

1. Preheat air fryer to 330°F.
2. In a medium bowl, stir together flour, sugar, baking powder, and salt.
3. In a separate bowl, combine oil, egg, and milk and mix well.
4. Add egg mixture to dry ingredients and stir just until moistened.
5. Gently stir in blueberries.
6. Spoon batter evenly into muffin cups.
7. Place 4 muffin cups in air fryer basket and bake at 330°F for 14 minutes or until tops spring back when touched lightly.
8. Repeat previous step to cook remaining muffins.

Fry Bread

Servings: 4
Cooking Time: 5 Minutes

Ingredients:

- 1 cup flour
- 2 teaspoons baking powder
- ¼ teaspoon salt
- ¼ cup lukewarm milk
- 1 teaspoon oil
- 2–3 tablespoons water
- oil for misting or cooking spray

Directions:

1. Stir together flour, baking powder, and salt. Gently mix in the milk and oil. Stir in 1 tablespoon water. If needed, add more water 1 tablespoon at a time until stiff dough forms. Dough shouldn't be sticky, so use only as much as you need.
2. Divide dough into 4 portions and shape into balls. Cover with a towel and let rest for 10minutes.
3. Preheat air fryer to 390°F.
4. Shape dough as desired:
5. a. Pat into 3-inch circles. This will make a thicker bread to eat plain or with a sprinkle of cinnamon or honey butter. You can cook all 4 at once.
6. b. Pat thinner into rectangles about 3 x 6 inches. This will create a thinner bread to serve as a base for dishes such as Indian tacos. The circular shape is more traditional, but rectangles allow you to cook 2 at a time in your air fryer basket.
7. Spray both sides of dough pieces with oil or cooking spray.
8. Place the 4 circles or 2 of the dough rectangles in the air fryer basket and cook at 390°F for 3minutes. Spray tops, turn, spray other side, and cook for 2 more minutes. If necessary, repeat to cook remaining bread.
9. Serve piping hot as is or allow to cool slightly and add toppings to create your own Native American tacos.

Breakfast Chimichangas

Servings: 4

Cooking Time: 8 Minutes

Ingredients:

- Four 8-inch flour tortillas
- ½ cup canned refried beans
- 1 cup scrambled eggs
- ½ cup grated cheddar or Monterey jack cheese
- 1 tablespoon vegetable oil
- 1 cup salsa

Directions:

1. Lay the flour tortillas out flat on a cutting board. In the center of each tortilla, spread 2 tablespoons refried beans. Next, add ¼ cup eggs and 2 tablespoons cheese to each tortilla.

2. To fold the tortillas, begin on the left side and fold to the center. Then fold the right side into the center. Next fold the bottom and top down and roll over to completely seal the chimichanga. Using a pastry brush or oil mister, brush the tops of the tortilla packages with oil.

3. Preheat the air fryer to 400°F for 4 minutes. Place the chimichangas into the air fryer basket, seam side down, and air fry for 4 minutes. Using tongs, turn over the chimichangas and cook for an additional 2 to 3 minutes or until light golden brown.

Hole In One

Servings: 1

Cooking Time: 7 Minutes

Ingredients:

- 1 slice bread
- 1 teaspoon soft butter
- 1 egg
- salt and pepper
- 1 tablespoon shredded Cheddar cheese
- 2 teaspoons diced ham

Directions:

1. Place a 6 x 6-inch baking dish inside air fryer basket and preheat fryer to 330°F.

2. Using a 2½-inch-diameter biscuit cutter, cut a hole in center of bread slice.

3. Spread softened butter on both sides of bread.

4. Lay bread slice in baking dish and crack egg into the hole. Sprinkle egg with salt and pepper to taste.

5. Cook for 5minutes.

6. Turn toast over and top it with shredded cheese and diced ham.

7. Cook for 2 more minutes or until yolk is done to your liking.

Poultry Recipes

Asian Meatball Tacos

Servings: 4
Cooking Time: 10 Minutes
Ingredients:

- 1 pound lean ground turkey
- 3 tablespoons soy sauce
- 1 tablespoon brown sugar
- ½ teaspoon onion powder
- ½ teaspoon garlic powder
- 1 tablespoon sesame seeds
- 1 English cucumber
- 4 radishes
- 2 tablespoons white wine vinegar
- 1 lime, juiced and divided
- 1 tablespoon avocado oil
- Salt, to taste
- ½ cup Greek yogurt
- 1 to 3 teaspoons Sriracha, based on desired spiciness
- 1 cup shredded cabbage
- ¼ cup chopped cilantro
- Eight 6-inch flour tortillas

Directions:

1. Preheat the air fryer to 360°F.
2. In a large bowl, mix the ground turkey, soy sauce, brown sugar, onion powder, garlic powder, and sesame seeds. Form the meat into 1-inch meatballs and place in the air fryer basket. Cook for 5 minutes, shake the basket, and cook another 5 minutes. Using a food thermometer, make sure the internal temperature of the meatballs is 165°F.
3. Meanwhile, dice the cucumber and radishes and place in a medium bowl. Add the white wine vinegar, 1 teaspoon of the lime juice, and the avocado oil, and stir to coat. Season with salt to desired taste.
4. In a large bowl, mix the Greek yogurt, Sriracha, and the remaining lime juice, and stir. Add in the cabbage and cilantro; toss well to create a slaw.
5. In a heavy skillet, heat the tortillas over medium heat for 1 to 2 minutes on each side, or until warmed.
6. To serve, place a tortilla on a plate, top with 5 meatballs, then with cucumber and radish salad, and finish with 2 tablespoons of cabbage slaw.

Lemon Sage Roast Chicken

Servings: 4
Cooking Time: 60 Minutes
Ingredients:

- 1 (4-pound) chicken
- 1 bunch sage, divided
- 1 lemon, zest and juice
- salt and freshly ground black pepper

Directions:

1. Preheat the air fryer to 350°F and pour a little water into the bottom of the air fryer drawer. (This will help prevent the grease that drips into the bottom drawer from burning and smoking.)
2. Run your fingers between the skin and flesh of the chicken breasts and thighs. Push a couple of sage leaves up underneath the skin of the chicken on each breast and each thigh.
3. Push some of the lemon zest up under the skin of the chicken next to the sage. Sprinkle some of the zest inside the chicken cavity, and reserve any leftover zest. Squeeze the lemon juice all over the chicken and in the cavity as well.

4. Season the chicken, inside and out, with the salt and freshly ground black pepper. Set a few sage leaves aside for the final garnish. Crumple up the remaining sage leaves and push them into the cavity of the chicken, along with one of the squeezed lemon halves.

5. Place the chicken breast side up into the air fryer basket and air-fry for 20 minutes at 350°F. Flip the chicken over so that it is breast side down and continue to air-fry for another 20 minutes. Return the chicken to breast side up and finish air-frying for 20 more minutes. The internal temperature of the chicken should register 165°F in the thickest part of the thigh when fully cooked. Remove the chicken from the air fryer and let it rest on a cutting board for at least 5 minutes.

6. Cut the rested chicken into pieces, sprinkle with the reserved lemon zest and garnish with the reserved sage leaves.

Peachy Chicken Chunks With Cherries

Servings: 4

Cooking Time: 16 Minutes

Ingredients:

- ⅓ cup peach preserves
- 1 teaspoon ground rosemary
- ½ teaspoon black pepper
- ½ teaspoon salt
- ½ teaspoon marjoram
- 1 teaspoon light olive oil
- 1 pound boneless chicken breasts, cut in 1½-inch chunks
- oil for misting or cooking spray
- 10-ounce package frozen unsweetened dark cherries, thawed and drained

Directions:

1. In a medium bowl, mix together peach preserves, rosemary, pepper, salt, marjoram, and olive oil.

2. Stir in chicken chunks and toss to coat well with the preserve mixture.

3. Spray air fryer basket with oil or cooking spray and lay chicken chunks in basket.

4. Cook at 390°F for 7minutes. Stir. Cook for 8 more minutes or until chicken juices run clear.

5. When chicken has cooked through, scatter the cherries over and cook for additional minute to heat cherries.

Pecan Turkey Cutlets

Servings: 4

Cooking Time: 12 Minutes

Ingredients:

- ¾ cup panko breadcrumbs
- ¼ teaspoon salt
- ¼ teaspoon pepper
- ¼ teaspoon dry mustard
- ¼ teaspoon poultry seasoning
- ½ cup pecans
- ¼ cup cornstarch
- 1 egg, beaten
- 1 pound turkey cutlets, ½-inch thick
- salt and pepper
- oil for misting or cooking spray

Directions:

1. Place the panko crumbs, ¼ teaspoon salt, ¼ teaspoon pepper, mustard, and poultry seasoning in food processor. Process until crumbs are finely crushed. Add pecans and process in short pulses just until nuts are finely chopped. Go easy so you don't overdo it!

2. Preheat air fryer to 360°F.

3. Place cornstarch in one shallow dish and beaten egg in another. Transfer coating mixture from food processor into a third shallow dish.

4. Sprinkle turkey cutlets with salt and pepper to taste.

5. Dip cutlets in cornstarch and shake off excess. Then dip in beaten egg and roll in crumbs, pressing to coat well. Spray both sides with oil or cooking spray.

6. Place 2 cutlets in air fryer basket in a single layer and cook for 12 minutes or until juices run clear.

7. Repeat step 6 to cook remaining cutlets.

Chicken Rochambeau

Servings: 4

Cooking Time: 20 Minutes

Ingredients:

- 1 tablespoon butter
- 4 chicken tenders, cut in half crosswise
- salt and pepper
- ¼ cup flour
- oil for misting
- 4 slices ham, ¼- to ⅜-inches thick and large enough to cover an English muffin
- 2 English muffins, split
- Sauce
- 2 tablespoons butter
- ½ cup chopped green onions
- ½ cup chopped mushrooms
- 2 tablespoons flour
- 1 cup chicken broth
- ¼ teaspoon garlic powder
- 1½ teaspoons Worcestershire sauce

Directions:

1. Place 1 tablespoon of butter in air fryer baking pan and cook at 390°F for 2minutes to melt.

2. Sprinkle chicken tenders with salt and pepper to taste, then roll in the ¼ cup of flour.

3. Place chicken in baking pan, turning pieces to coat with melted butter.

4. Cook at 390°F for 5minutes. Turn chicken pieces over, and spray tops lightly with olive oil. Cook 5minutes longer or until juices run clear. The chicken will not brown.

5. While chicken is cooking, make the sauce: In a medium saucepan, melt the 2 tablespoons of butter.

6. Add onions and mushrooms and sauté until tender, about 3minutes.

7. Stir in the flour. Gradually add broth, stirring constantly until you have a smooth gravy.

8. Add garlic powder and Worcestershire sauce and simmer on low heat until sauce thickens, about 5minutes.

9. When chicken is cooked, remove baking pan from air fryer and set aside.

10. Place ham slices directly into air fryer basket and cook at 390°F for 5minutes or until hot and beginning to sizzle a little. Remove and set aside on top of the chicken for now.

11. Place the English muffin halves in air fryer basket and cook at 390°F for 1 minute.

12. Open air fryer and place a ham slice on top of each English muffin half. Stack 2 pieces of chicken on top of each ham slice. Cook at 390°F for 1 to 2minutes to heat through.

13. Place each English muffin stack on a serving plate and top with plenty of sauce.

Tortilla Crusted Chicken Breast

Servings: 2
Cooking Time: 12 Minutes

Ingredients:

- ⅓ cup flour
- 1 teaspoon salt
- 1½ teaspoons chili powder
- 1 teaspoon ground cumin
- freshly ground black pepper
- 1 egg, beaten
- ¾ cup coarsely crushed yellow corn tortilla chips
- 2 (3- to 4-ounce) boneless chicken breasts
- vegetable oil
- ½ cup salsa
- ½ cup crumbled queso fresco
- fresh cilantro leaves
- sour cream or guacamole (optional)

Directions:

1. Set up a dredging station with three shallow dishes. Combine the flour, salt, chili powder, cumin and black pepper in the first shallow dish. Beat the egg in the second shallow dish. Place the crushed tortilla chips in the third shallow dish.
2. Dredge the chicken in the spiced flour, covering all sides of the breast. Then dip the chicken into the egg, coating the chicken completely. Finally, place the chicken into the tortilla chips and press the chips onto the chicken to make sure they adhere to all sides of the breast. Spray the coated chicken breasts on both sides with vegetable oil.
3. Preheat the air fryer to 380°F.
4. Air-fry the chicken for 6 minutes. Then turn the chicken breasts over and air-fry for another 6 minutes. (Increase the cooking time if you are using chicken breasts larger than 3 to 4 ounces.)
5. When the chicken has finished cooking, serve each breast with a little salsa, the crumbled queso fresco and cilantro as the finishing touch. Serve some sour cream and/or guacamole at the table, if desired.

Chicken Cordon Bleu

Servings: 2
Cooking Time: 16 Minutes

Ingredients:

- 2 boneless, skinless chicken breasts
- ¼ teaspoon salt
- 2 teaspoons Dijon mustard
- 2 ounces deli ham
- 2 ounces Swiss, fontina, or Gruyère cheese
- ⅓ cup all-purpose flour
- 1 egg
- ½ cup breadcrumbs

Directions:

1. Pat the chicken breasts with a paper towel. Season the chicken with the salt. Pound the chicken breasts to 1½ inches thick. Create a pouch by slicing the side of each chicken breast. Spread 1 teaspoon Dijon mustard inside the pouch of each chicken breast. Wrap a 1-ounce slice of ham around a 1-ounce slice of cheese and place into the pouch. Repeat with the remaining ham and cheese.
2. In a medium bowl, place the flour.
3. In a second bowl, whisk the egg.
4. In a third bowl, place the breadcrumbs.
5. Dredge the chicken in the flour and shake off the excess. Next, dip the chicken into the egg and then in the breadcrumbs. Set the chicken on a plate and repeat with the remaining chicken piece.
6. Preheat the air fryer to 360°F.
7. Place the chicken in the air fryer basket and spray liberally with cooking spray. Cook for 8

minutes, turn the chicken breasts over, and liberally spray with cooking spray again; cook another 6 minutes. Once golden brown, check for an internal temperature of 165°F.

Chicken Tikka

Servings: 4
Cooking Time: 15 Minutes
Ingredients:
- ¼ cup plain Greek yogurt
- 1 clove garlic, minced
- 1 tablespoon ketchup
- 1 tablespoon extra-virgin olive oil
- 1 tablespoon lemon juice
- ½ teaspoon salt
- ½ teaspoon ground cumin
- ½ teaspoon paprika
- ¼ teaspoon ground cinnamon
- ½ teaspoon ground black pepper
- ½ teaspoon cayenne pepper
- 1 pound boneless, skinless chicken thighs

Directions:
1. In a large bowl, stir together the yogurt, garlic, ketchup, olive oil, lemon juice, salt, cumin, paprika, cinnamon, black pepper, and cayenne pepper until combined.
2. Add the chicken thighs to the bow and fold the yogurt-spice mixture over the chicken thighs until they're covered with the marinade. Cover with plastic wrap and place in the refrigerator for 30 minutes.
3. When ready to cook the chicken, remove from the refrigerator and preheat the air fryer to 370°F.
4. Liberally spray the air fryer basket with olive oil mist. Place the chicken thighs into the air fryer basket, leaving space between the thighs to turn.
5. Cook for 10 minutes, turn the chicken thighs, and cook another 5 minutes (or until the internal temperature reaches 165°F).
6. Remove the chicken from the air fryer and serve warm with desired sides.

Southern-fried Chicken Livers

Servings: 4
Cooking Time: 12 Minutes
Ingredients:
- 2 eggs
- 2 tablespoons water
- ¾ cup flour
- 1½ cups panko breadcrumbs
- ½ cup plain breadcrumbs
- 1 teaspoon salt
- ½ teaspoon black pepper
- 20 ounces chicken livers, salted to taste
- oil for misting or cooking spray

Directions:
1. Beat together eggs and water in a shallow dish. Place the flour in a separate shallow dish.
2. In the bowl of a food processor, combine the panko, plain breadcrumbs, salt, and pepper. Process until well mixed and panko crumbs are finely crushed. Place crumbs in a third shallow dish.
3. Dip livers in flour, then egg wash, and then roll in panko mixture to coat well with crumbs.
4. Spray both sides of livers with oil or cooking spray. Cooking in two batches, place livers in air fryer basket in single layer.
5. Cook at 390°F for 7minutes. Spray livers, turn over, and spray again. Cook for 5 more minutes, until done inside and coating is golden brown.
6. Repeat to cook remaining livers.

Jerk Turkey Meatballs

Servings: 7

Cooking Time: 8 Minutes

Ingredients:

- 1 pound lean ground turkey
- ¼ cup chopped onion
- 1 teaspoon minced garlic
- ½ teaspoon dried thyme
- ¼ teaspoon ground cinnamon
- 1 teaspoon cayenne pepper
- ½ teaspoon paprika
- ½ teaspoon salt
- ⅛ teaspoon black pepper
- ¼ teaspoon red pepper flakes
- 2 teaspoons brown sugar
- 1 large egg, whisked
- ⅓ cup panko breadcrumbs
- 2⅓ cups cooked brown Jasmine rice
- 2 green onions, chopped
- ¾ cup sweet onion dressing

Directions:

1. Preheat the air fryer to 350°F.

2. In a medium bowl, mix the ground turkey with the onion, garlic, thyme, cinnamon, cayenne pepper, paprika, salt, pepper, red pepper flakes, and brown sugar. Add the whisked egg and stir in the breadcrumbs until the turkey starts to hold together.

3. Using a 1-ounce scoop, portion the turkey into meatballs. You should get about 28 meatballs.

4. Spray the air fryer basket with olive oil spray.

5. Place the meatballs into the air fryer basket and cook for 5 minutes, shake the basket, and cook another 2 to 4 minutes (or until the internal temperature of the meatballs reaches 165°F).

6. Remove the meatballs from the basket and repeat for the remaining meatballs.

7. Serve warm over a bed of rice with chopped green onions and spicy Caribbean jerk dressing.

Crispy Duck With Cherry Sauce

Servings: 2

Cooking Time: 33 Minutes

Ingredients:

- 1 whole duck (up to 5 pounds), split in half, back and rib bones removed
- 1 teaspoon olive oil
- salt and freshly ground black pepper
- Cherry Sauce:
- 1 tablespoon butter
- 1 shallot, minced
- ½ cup sherry
- ¾ cup cherry preserves 1 cup chicken stock
- 1 teaspoon white wine vinegar
- 1 teaspoon fresh thyme leaves
- salt and freshly ground black pepper

Directions:

1. Preheat the air fryer to 400°F.

2. Trim some of the fat from the duck. Rub olive oil on the duck and season with salt and pepper. Place the duck halves in the air fryer basket, breast side up and facing the center of the basket.

3. Air-fry the duck for 20 minutes. Turn the duck over and air-fry for another 6 minutes.

4. While duck is air-frying, make the cherry sauce. Melt the butter in a large sauté pan. Add the shallot and sauté until it is just starting to brown – about 2 to 3 minutes. Add the sherry and deglaze the pan by scraping up any brown bits from the bottom of the pan. Simmer the liquid for a few minutes, until it has reduced by half. Add the cherry preserves, chicken stock and white wine vinegar. Whisk well to combine all the ingredients. Simmer the sauce until it

thickens and coats the back of a spoon – about 5 to 7 minutes. Season with salt and pepper and stir in the fresh thyme leaves.

5. When the air fryer timer goes off, spoon some cherry sauce over the duck and continue to air-fry at 400°F for 4 more minutes. Then, turn the duck halves back over so that the breast side is facing up. Spoon more cherry sauce over the top of the duck, covering the skin completely. Air-fry for 3 more minutes and then remove the duck to a plate to rest for a few minutes.

6. Serve the duck in halves, or cut each piece in half again for a smaller serving. Spoon any additional sauce over the duck or serve it on the side.

Sweet Chili Spiced Chicken

Servings: 4
Cooking Time: 43 Minutes
Ingredients:
- Spice Rub:
- 2 tablespoons brown sugar
- 2 tablespoons paprika
- 1 teaspoon dry mustard powder
- 1 teaspoon chili powder
- 2 tablespoons coarse sea salt or kosher salt
- 2 teaspoons coarsely ground black pepper
- 1 tablespoon vegetable oil
- 1 (3½-pound) chicken, cut into 8 pieces

Directions:
1. Prepare the spice rub by combining the brown sugar, paprika, mustard powder, chili powder, salt and pepper. Rub the oil all over the chicken pieces and then rub the spice mix onto the chicken, covering completely. This is done very easily in a zipper sealable bag. You can do this ahead of time and let the chicken marinate in the refrigerator, or just proceed with cooking right away.

2. Preheat the air fryer to 370°F.

3. Air-fry the chicken in two batches. Place the two chicken thighs and two drumsticks into the air fryer basket. Air-fry at 370°F for 10 minutes. Then, gently turn the chicken pieces over and air-fry for another 10 minutes. Remove the chicken pieces and let them rest on a plate while you cook the chicken breasts. Air-fry the chicken breasts, skin side down for 8 minutes. Turn the chicken breasts over and air-fry for another 12 minutes.

4. Lower the temperature of the air fryer to 340°F. Place the first batch of chicken on top of the second batch already in the basket and air-fry for a final 3 minutes.

5. Let the chicken rest for 5 minutes and serve warm with some mashed potatoes and a green salad or vegetables.

Spicy Black Bean Turkey Burgers With Cumin-avocado Spread

Servings: 2
Cooking Time: 20 Minutes
Ingredients:
- 1 cup canned black beans, drained and rinsed
- ¾ pound lean ground turkey
- 2 tablespoons minced red onion
- 1 Jalapeño pepper, seeded and minced
- 2 tablespoons plain breadcrumbs
- ½ teaspoon chili powder
- ¼ teaspoon cayenne pepper
- salt, to taste
- olive or vegetable oil
- 2 slices pepper jack cheese
- toasted burger rolls, sliced tomatoes, lettuce leaves

- Cumin-Avocado Spread:
- 1 ripe avocado
- juice of 1 lime
- 1 teaspoon ground cumin
- ½ teaspoon salt
- 1 tablespoon chopped fresh cilantro
- freshly ground black pepper

Directions:

1. Place the black beans in a large bowl and smash them slightly with the back of a fork. Add the ground turkey, red onion, Jalapeño pepper, breadcrumbs, chili powder and cayenne pepper. Season with salt. Mix with your hands to combine all the ingredients and then shape them into 2 patties. Brush both sides of the burger patties with a little olive or vegetable oil.

2. Preheat the air fryer to 380°F.

3. Transfer the burgers to the air fryer basket and air-fry for 20 minutes, flipping them over halfway through the cooking process. Top the burgers with the pepper jack cheese (securing the slices to the burgers with a toothpick) for the last 2 minutes of the cooking process.

4. While the burgers are cooking, make the cumin avocado spread. Place the avocado, lime juice, cumin and salt in food processor and process until smooth. (For a chunkier spread, you can mash this by hand in a bowl.) Stir in the cilantro and season with freshly ground black pepper. Chill the spread until you are ready to serve.

5. When the burgers have finished cooking, remove them from the air fryer and let them rest on a plate, covered gently with aluminum foil. Brush a little olive oil on the insides of the burger rolls. Place the rolls, cut side up, into the air fryer basket and air-fry at 400°F for 1 minute to toast and warm them.

6. Spread the cumin-avocado spread on the rolls and build your burgers with lettuce and sliced tomatoes and any other ingredient you like. Serve warm with a side of sweet potato fries.

Thai Turkey And Zucchini Meatballs

Servings: 4

Cooking Time: 12 Minutes

Ingredients:

- 1½ cups grated zucchini,
- squeezed dry in a clean kitchen towel (about 1 large zucchini)
- 3 scallions, finely chopped
- 2 cloves garlic, minced
- 1 tablespoon grated fresh ginger
- 1 tablespoon finely chopped fresh cilantro
- zest of 1 lime
- 1 teaspoon salt
- freshly ground black pepper
- 1½ pounds ground turkey (a mix of light and dark meat)
- 2 eggs, lightly beaten
- 1 cup Thai sweet chili sauce (spring roll sauce)
- lime wedges, for serving

Directions:

1. Combine the zucchini, scallions, garlic, ginger, cilantro, lime zest, salt, pepper, ground turkey and eggs in a bowl and mix the ingredients together. Gently shape the mixture into 24 balls, about the size of golf balls.

2. Preheat the air fryer to 380°F.

3. Working in batches, air-fry the meatballs for 12 minutes, turning the meatballs over halfway through the cooking time. As soon as the meatballs have finished cooking, toss them in a bowl with the Thai sweet chili sauce to coat.

4. Serve the meatballs over rice noodles or white rice with the remaining Thai sweet chili sauce and lime wedges to squeeze over the top.

Sweet-and-sour Chicken

Servings: 6
Cooking Time: 10 Minutes
Ingredients:
- 1 cup pineapple juice
- 1 cup plus 3 tablespoons cornstarch, divided
- ¼ cup sugar
- ¼ cup ketchup
- ¼ cup apple cider vinegar
- 2 tablespoons soy sauce or tamari
- 1 teaspoon garlic powder, divided
- ¼ cup flour
- 1 tablespoon sesame seeds
- ½ teaspoon salt
- ¼ teaspoon ground black pepper
- 2 large eggs
- 2 pounds chicken breasts, cut into 1-inch cubes
- 1 red bell pepper, cut into 1-inch pieces
- 1 carrot, sliced into ¼-inch-thick rounds

Directions:
1. In a medium saucepan, whisk together the pineapple juice, 3 tablespoons of the cornstarch, the sugar, the ketchup, the apple cider vinegar, the soy sauce or tamari, and ½ teaspoon of the garlic powder. Cook over medium-low heat, whisking occasionally as the sauce thickens, about 6 minutes. Stir and set aside while preparing the chicken.
2. Preheat the air fryer to 370°F.
3. In a medium bowl, place the remaining 1 cup of cornstarch, the flour, the sesame seeds, the salt, the remaining ½ teaspoon of garlic powder, and the pepper.

4. In a second medium bowl, whisk the eggs.
5. Working in batches, place the cubed chicken in the cornstarch mixture to lightly coat; then dip it into the egg mixture, and return it to the cornstarch mixture. Shake off the excess and place the coated chicken in the air fryer basket. Spray with cooking spray and cook for 5 minutes, shake the basket, and spray with more cooking spray. Cook an additional 3 to 5 minutes, or until completely cooked and golden brown.
6. On the last batch of chicken, add the bell pepper and carrot to the basket and cook with the chicken.
7. Place the cooked chicken and vegetables into a serving bowl and toss with the sweet-and-sour sauce to serve.

Nacho Chicken Fries

Servings: 4
Cooking Time: 7 Minutes
Ingredients:
- 1 pound chicken tenders
- salt
- ¼ cup flour
- 2 eggs
- ¾ cup panko breadcrumbs
- ¾ cup crushed organic nacho cheese tortilla chips
- oil for misting or cooking spray
- Seasoning Mix
- 1 tablespoon chili powder
- 1 teaspoon ground cumin
- ½ teaspoon garlic powder
- ½ teaspoon onion powder

Directions:
1. Stir together all seasonings in a small cup and set aside.

2. Cut chicken tenders in half crosswise, then cut into strips no wider than about ½ inch.

3. Preheat air fryer to 390°F.

4. Salt chicken to taste. Place strips in large bowl and sprinkle with 1 tablespoon of the seasoning mix. Stir well to distribute seasonings.

5. Add flour to chicken and stir well to coat all sides.

6. Beat eggs together in a shallow dish.

7. In a second shallow dish, combine the panko, crushed chips, and the remaining 2 teaspoons of seasoning mix.

8. Dip chicken strips in eggs, then roll in crumbs. Mist with oil or cooking spray.

9. Chicken strips will cook best if done in two batches. They can be crowded and overlapping a little but not stacked in double or triple layers.

10. Cook for 4minutes. Shake basket, mist with oil, and cook 3 moreminutes, until chicken juices run clear and outside is crispy.

11. Repeat step 10 to cook remaining chicken fries.

Chicken Chunks

Servings: 4
Cooking Time: 10 Minutes
Ingredients:
- 1 pound chicken tenders cut in large chunks, about 1½ inches
- salt and pepper
- ½ cup cornstarch
- 2 eggs, beaten
- 1 cup panko breadcrumbs
- oil for misting or cooking spray

Directions:
1. Season chicken chunks to your liking with salt and pepper.

2. Dip chicken chunks in cornstarch. Then dip in egg and shake off excess. Then roll in panko crumbs to coat well.

3. Spray all sides of chicken chunks with oil or cooking spray.

4. Place chicken in air fryer basket in single layer and cook at 390°F for 5minutes. Spray with oil, turn chunks over, and spray other side.

5. Cook for an additional 5minutes or until chicken juices run clear and outside is golden brown.

6. Repeat steps 4 and 5 to cook remaining chicken.

Teriyaki Chicken Legs

Servings: 2
Cooking Time: 20 Minutes
Ingredients:
- 4 tablespoons teriyaki sauce
- 1 tablespoon orange juice
- 1 teaspoon smoked paprika
- 4 chicken legs
- cooking spray

Directions:
1. Mix together the teriyaki sauce, orange juice, and smoked paprika. Brush on all sides of chicken legs.

2. Spray air fryer basket with nonstick cooking spray and place chicken in basket.

3. Cook at 360°F for 6minutes. Turn and baste with sauce. Cook for 6 moreminutes, turn and baste. Cook for 8 minutes more, until juices run clear when chicken is pierced with a fork.

Buttermilk-fried Drumsticks

Servings: 2
Cooking Time: 25 Minutes

Ingredients:
- 1 egg
- ½ cup buttermilk
- ¾ cup self-rising flour
- ¾ cup seasoned panko breadcrumbs
- 1 teaspoon salt
- ¼ teaspoon ground black pepper (to mix into coating)
- 4 chicken drumsticks, skin on
- oil for misting or cooking spray

Directions:
1. Beat together egg and buttermilk in shallow dish.
2. In a second shallow dish, combine the flour, panko crumbs, salt, and pepper.
3. Sprinkle chicken legs with additional salt and pepper to taste.
4. Dip legs in buttermilk mixture, then roll in panko mixture, pressing in crumbs to make coating stick. Mist with oil or cooking spray.
5. Spray air fryer basket with cooking spray.
6. Cook drumsticks at 360°F for 10minutes. Turn pieces over and cook an additional 10minutes.
7. Turn pieces to check for browning. If you have any white spots that haven't begun to brown, spritz them with oil or cooking spray. Continue cooking for 5 more minutes or until crust is golden brown and juices run clear. Larger, meatier drumsticks will take longer to cook than small ones.

Chicken Parmesan

Servings: 4
Cooking Time: 11 Minutes
Ingredients:
- 4 chicken tenders
- Italian seasoning
- salt
- ¼ cup cornstarch
- ½ cup Italian salad dressing
- ¼ cup panko breadcrumbs
- ¼ cup grated Parmesan cheese, plus more for serving
- oil for misting or cooking spray
- 8 ounces spaghetti, cooked
- 1 24-ounce jar marinara sauce

Directions:
1. Pound chicken tenders with meat mallet or rolling pin until about ¼-inch thick.
2. Sprinkle both sides with Italian seasoning and salt to taste.
3. Place cornstarch and salad dressing in 2 separate shallow dishes.
4. In a third shallow dish, mix together the panko crumbs and Parmesan cheese.
5. Dip flattened chicken in cornstarch, then salad dressing. Dip in the panko mixture, pressing into the chicken so the coating sticks well.
6. Spray both sides with oil or cooking spray. Place in air fryer basket in single layer.
7. Cook at 390°F for 5minutes. Spray with oil again, turning chicken to coat both sides. See tip about turning.
8. Cook for an additional 6 minutes or until chicken juices run clear and outside is browned.
9. While chicken is cooking, heat marinara sauce and stir into cooked spaghetti.
10. To serve, divide spaghetti with sauce among 4 dinner plates, and top each with a fried chicken tender. Pass additional Parmesan at the table for those who want extra cheese.

Buffalo Egg Rolls

Servings: 8
Cooking Time: 9 Minutes Per Batch

Ingredients:

- 1 teaspoon water
- 1 tablespoon cornstarch
- 1 egg
- 2½ cups cooked chicken, diced or shredded (see opposite page)
- ⅓ cup chopped green onion
- ⅓ cup diced celery
- ⅓ cup buffalo wing sauce
- 8 egg roll wraps
- oil for misting or cooking spray
- Blue Cheese Dip
- 3 ounces cream cheese, softened
- ⅓ cup blue cheese, crumbled
- 1 teaspoon Worcestershire sauce
- ¼ teaspoon garlic powder
- ¼ cup buttermilk (or sour cream)

Directions:

1. Mix water and cornstarch in a small bowl until dissolved. Add egg, beat well, and set aside.
2. In a medium size bowl, mix together chicken, green onion, celery, and buffalo wing sauce.
3. Divide chicken mixture evenly among 8 egg roll wraps, spooning ½ inch from one edge.
4. Moisten all edges of each wrap with beaten egg wash.
5. Fold the short ends over filling, then roll up tightly and press to seal edges.
6. Brush outside of wraps with egg wash, then spritz with oil or cooking spray.
7. Place 4 egg rolls in air fryer basket.
8. Cook at 390°F for 9minutes or until outside is brown and crispy.
9. While the rolls are cooking, prepare the Blue Cheese Dip. With a fork, mash together cream cheese and blue cheese.
10. Stir in remaining ingredients.
11. Dip should be just thick enough to slightly cling to egg rolls. If too thick, stir in buttermilk or milk 1 tablespoon at a time until you reach the desired consistency.
12. Cook remaining 4 egg rolls as in steps 7 and 8.
13. Serve while hot with Blue Cheese Dip, more buffalo wing sauce, or both.

Chicken Chimichangas

Servings: 4

Cooking Time: 10 Minutes

Ingredients:

- 2 cups cooked chicken, shredded
- 2 tablespoons chopped green chiles
- ½ teaspoon oregano
- ½ teaspoon cumin
- ½ teaspoon onion powder
- ¼ teaspoon garlic powder
- salt and pepper
- 8 flour tortillas (6- or 7-inch diameter)
- oil for misting or cooking spray
- Chimichanga Sauce
- 2 tablespoons butter
- 2 tablespoons flour
- 1 cup chicken broth
- ¼ cup light sour cream
- ¼ teaspoon salt
- 2 ounces Pepper Jack or Monterey Jack cheese, shredded

Directions:

1. Make the sauce by melting butter in a saucepan over medium-low heat. Stir in flour until smooth and slightly bubbly. Gradually add broth, stirring constantly until smooth. Cook and stir 1 minute, until the mixture slightly thickens. Remove from heat and stir in sour cream and salt. Set aside.

2. In a medium bowl, mix together the chicken, chiles, oregano, cumin, onion powder, garlic, salt, and pepper. Stir in 3 to 4 tablespoons of the sauce, using just enough to make the filling moist but not soupy.

3. Divide filling among the 8 tortillas. Place filling down the center of tortilla, stopping about 1 inch from edges. Fold one side of tortilla over filling, fold the two sides in, and then roll up. Mist all sides with oil or cooking spray.

4. Place chimichangas in air fryer basket seam side down. To fit more into the basket, you can stand them on their sides with the seams against the sides of the basket.

5. Cook at 360°F for 10 minutes or until heated through and crispy brown outside.

6. Add the shredded cheese to the remaining sauce. Stir over low heat, warming just until the cheese melts. Don't boil or sour cream may curdle.

7. Drizzle the sauce over the chimichangas.

Pickle Brined Fried Chicken

Servings: 4
Cooking Time: 47 Minutes
Ingredients:
- 4 bone-in, skin-on chicken legs, cut into drumsticks and thighs (about 3½ pounds)
- pickle juice from a 24-ounce jar of kosher dill pickles
- ½ cup flour
- salt and freshly ground black pepper
- 2 eggs
- 1 cup fine breadcrumbs
- 1 teaspoon salt
- 1 teaspoon freshly ground black pepper
- ½ teaspoon ground paprika
- ⅛ teaspoon ground cayenne pepper
- vegetable or canola oil in a spray bottle

Directions:

1. Place the chicken in a shallow dish and pour the pickle juice over the top. Cover and transfer the chicken to the refrigerator to brine in the pickle juice for 3 to 8 hours.

2. When you are ready to cook, remove the chicken from the refrigerator to let it come to room temperature while you set up a dredging station. Place the flour in a shallow dish and season well with salt and freshly ground black pepper. Whisk the eggs in a second shallow dish. In a third shallow dish, combine the breadcrumbs, salt, pepper, paprika and cayenne pepper.

3. Preheat the air fryer to 370°F.

4. Remove the chicken from the pickle brine and gently dry it with a clean kitchen towel. Dredge each piece of chicken in the flour, then dip it into the egg mixture, and finally press it into the breadcrumb mixture to coat all sides of the chicken. Place the breaded chicken on a plate or baking sheet and spray each piece all over with vegetable oil.

5. Air-fry the chicken in two batches. Place two chicken thighs and two drumsticks into the air fryer basket. Air-fry for 10 minutes. Then, gently turn the chicken pieces over and air-fry for another 10 minutes. Remove the chicken pieces and let them rest on plate – do not cover. Repeat with the second batch of chicken, air-frying for 20 minutes, turning the chicken over halfway through.

6. Lower the temperature of the air fryer to 340°F. Place the first batch of chicken on top of the second batch already in the basket and air-fry for an additional 7 minutes. Serve warm and enjoy.

Crispy Fried Onion Chicken Breasts

Servings: 2

Cooking Time: 13 Minutes

Ingredients:

- ¼ cup all-purpose flour*
- salt and freshly ground black pepper
- 1 egg
- 2 tablespoons Dijon mustard
- 1½ cups crispy fried onions (like French's®)
- ½ teaspoon paprika
- 2 (5-ounce) boneless, skinless chicken breasts
- vegetable or olive oil, in a spray bottle

Directions:

1. Preheat the air fryer to 380°F.

2. Set up a dredging station with three shallow dishes. Place the flour in the first shallow dish and season well with salt and freshly ground black pepper. Combine the egg and Dijon mustard in a second shallow dish and whisk until smooth. Place the fried onions in a sealed bag and using a rolling pin, crush them into coarse crumbs. Combine these crumbs with the paprika in the third shallow dish.

3. Dredge the chicken breasts in the flour. Shake off any excess flour and dip them into the egg mixture. Let any excess egg drip off. Then coat both sides of the chicken breasts with the crispy onions. Press the crumbs onto the chicken breasts with your hands to make sure they are well adhered.

4. Spray or brush the bottom of the air fryer basket with oil. Transfer the chicken breasts to the air fryer basket and air-fry at 380°F for 13 minutes, turning the chicken over halfway through the cooking time.

5. Serve immediately.

Chicken Souvlaki Gyros

Servings: 4

Cooking Time: 18 Minutes

Ingredients:

- ¼ cup extra-virgin olive oil
- 1 clove garlic, crushed
- 1 tablespoon Italian seasoning
- ½ teaspoon paprika
- ½ lemon, sliced
- ¼ teaspoon salt
- 1 pound boneless, skinless chicken breasts
- 4 whole-grain pita breads
- 1 cup shredded lettuce
- ½ cup chopped tomatoes
- ¼ cup chopped red onion
- ¼ cup cucumber yogurt sauce

Directions:

1. In a large resealable plastic bag, combine the olive oil, garlic, Italian seasoning, paprika, lemon, and salt. Add the chicken to the bag and secure shut. Vigorously shake until all the ingredients are combined. Set in the fridge for 2 hours to marinate.

2. When ready to cook, preheat the air fryer to 360°F.

3. Liberally spray the air fryer basket with olive oil mist. Remove the chicken from the bag and discard the leftover marinade. Place the chicken into the air fryer basket, allowing enough room between the chicken breasts to flip.

4. Cook for 10 minutes, flip, and cook another 8 minutes.

5. Remove the chicken from the air fryer basket when it has cooked (or the internal temperature of the chicken reaches 165°F). Let rest 5 minutes. Then thinly slice the chicken into strips.

6. Assemble the gyros by placing the pita bread on a flat surface and topping with chicken, lettuce, tomatoes, onion, and a drizzle of yogurt sauce.

7. Serve warm.

Spinach And Feta Stuffed Chicken Breasts

Servings: 4

Cooking Time: 27 Minutes

Ingredients:

- 1 (10-ounce) package frozen spinach, thawed and drained well
- 1 cup feta cheese, crumbled
- ½ teaspoon freshly ground black pepper
- 4 boneless chicken breasts
- salt and freshly ground black pepper
- 1 tablespoon olive oil

Directions:

1. Prepare the filling. Squeeze out as much liquid as possible from the thawed spinach. Rough chop the spinach and transfer it to a mixing bowl with the feta cheese and the freshly ground black pepper.

2. Prepare the chicken breast. Place the chicken breast on a cutting board and press down on the chicken breast with one hand to keep it stabilized. Make an incision about 1-inch long in the fattest side of the breast. Move the knife up and down inside the chicken breast, without poking through either the top or the bottom, or the other side of the breast. The inside pocket should be about 3-inches long, but the opening should only be about 1-inch wide. If this is too difficult, you can make the incision longer, but you will have to be more careful when cooking the chicken breast since this will expose more of the stuffing.

3. Once you have prepared the chicken breasts, use your fingers to stuff the filling into each pocket, spreading the mixture down as far as you can.

4. Preheat the air fryer to 380°F.

5. Lightly brush or spray the air fryer basket and the chicken breasts with olive oil. Transfer two of the stuffed chicken breasts to the air fryer. Air-fry for 12 minutes, turning the chicken breasts over halfway through the cooking time. Remove the chicken to a resting plate and air-fry the second two breasts for 12 minutes. Return the first batch of chicken to the air fryer with the second batch and air-fry for 3 more minutes. When the chicken is cooked, an instant read thermometer should register 165°F in the thickest part of the chicken, as well as in the stuffing.

6. Remove the chicken breasts and let them rest on a cutting board for 2 to 3 minutes. Slice the chicken on the bias and serve with the slices fanned out.

Teriyaki Chicken Drumsticks

Servings: 2

Cooking Time: 17 Minutes

Ingredients:

- 2 tablespoons soy sauce*
- ¼ cup dry sherry
- 1 tablespoon brown sugar
- 2 tablespoons water
- 1 tablespoon rice wine vinegar
- 1 clove garlic, crushed
- 1-inch fresh ginger, peeled and sliced
- pinch crushed red pepper flakes
- 4 to 6 bone-in, skin-on chicken drumsticks
- 1 tablespoon cornstarch
- fresh cilantro leaves

Directions:

1. Make the marinade by combining the soy sauce, dry sherry, brown sugar, water, rice vinegar, garlic, ginger and crushed red pepper flakes. Pour the marinade over the chicken legs, cover and let the chicken marinate for 1 to 4 hours in the refrigerator.

2. Preheat the air fryer to 380°F.

3. Transfer the chicken from the marinade to the air fryer basket, transferring any extra marinade to a small saucepan. Air-fry at 380°F for 8 minutes. Flip the chicken over and continue to air-fry for another 6 minutes, watching to make sure it doesn't brown too much.

4. While the chicken is cooking, bring the reserved marinade to a simmer on the stovetop. Dissolve the cornstarch in 2 tablespoons of water and stir this into the saucepan. Bring to a boil to thicken the sauce. Remove the garlic clove and slices of ginger from the sauce and set aside.

5. When the time is up on the air fryer, brush the thickened sauce on the chicken and air-fry for 3 more minutes. Remove the chicken from the air fryer and brush with the remaining sauce.

6. Serve over rice and sprinkle the cilantro leaves on top.

Quick Chicken For Filling

Servings: 2

Cooking Time: 8 Minutes

Ingredients:

- 1 pound chicken tenders, skinless and boneless
- ½ teaspoon ground cumin
- ½ teaspoon garlic powder
- cooking spray

Directions:

1. Sprinkle raw chicken tenders with seasonings.

2. Spray air fryer basket lightly with cooking spray to prevent sticking.

3. Place chicken in air fryer basket in single layer.

4. Cook at 390°F for 4minutes, turn chicken strips over, and cook for an additional 4minutes.

5. Test for doneness. Thick tenders may require an additional minute or two.

Air-fried Turkey Breast With Cherry Glaze

Servings: 6

Cooking Time: 54 Minutes

Ingredients:

- 1 (5-pound) turkey breast
- 2 teaspoons olive oil
- 1 teaspoon dried thyme
- ½ teaspoon dried sage
- 1 teaspoon salt
- ½ teaspoon freshly ground black pepper
- ½ cup cherry preserves
- 1 tablespoon chopped fresh thyme leaves
- 1 teaspoon soy sauce*
- freshly ground black pepper

Directions:

1. All turkeys are built differently, so depending on the turkey breast and how your butcher has prepared it, you may need to trim the bottom of the ribs in order to get the turkey to sit upright in the air fryer basket without touching the heating element. The key to this recipe is getting the right size turkey breast. Once you've managed that, the rest is easy, so make sure your turkey breast fits into the air fryer basket before you Preheat the air fryer.

2. Preheat the air fryer to 350°F.

3. Brush the turkey breast all over with the olive oil. Combine the thyme, sage, salt and pepper

and rub the outside of the turkey breast with the spice mixture.

4. Transfer the seasoned turkey breast to the air fryer basket, breast side up, and air-fry at 350°F for 25 minutes. Turn the turkey breast on its side and air-fry for another 12 minutes. Turn the turkey breast on the opposite side and air-fry for 12 more minutes. The internal temperature of the turkey breast should reach 165°F when fully cooked.

5. While the turkey is air-frying, make the glaze by combining the cherry preserves, fresh thyme, soy sauce and pepper in a small bowl. When the cooking time is up, return the turkey breast to an upright position and brush the glaze all over the turkey. Air-fry for a final 5 minutes, until the skin is nicely browned and crispy. Let the turkey rest, loosely tented with foil, for at least 5 minutes before slicing and serving.

Simple Buttermilk Fried Chicken

Servings: 4

Cooking Time: 27 Minutes

Ingredients:

- 1 (4-pound) chicken, cut into 8 pieces
- 2 cups buttermilk
- hot sauce (optional)
- 1½ cups flour*
- 2 teaspoons paprika
- 1 teaspoon salt
- freshly ground black pepper
- 2 eggs, lightly beaten
- vegetable oil, in a spray bottle

Directions:

1. Cut the chicken into 8 pieces and submerge them in the buttermilk and hot sauce, if using. A zipper-sealable plastic bag works well for this. Let the chicken soak in the buttermilk for at least one hour or even overnight in the refrigerator.

2. Set up a dredging station. Mix the flour, paprika, salt and black pepper in a clean zipper-sealable plastic bag. Whisk the eggs and place them in a shallow dish. Remove four pieces of chicken from the buttermilk and transfer them to the bag with the flour. Shake them around to coat on all sides. Remove the chicken from the flour, shaking off any excess flour, and dip them into the beaten egg. Return the chicken to the bag of seasoned flour and shake again. Set the coated chicken aside and repeat with the remaining four pieces of chicken.

3. Preheat the air fryer to 370°F.

4. Spray the chicken on all sides with the vegetable oil and then transfer one batch to the air fryer basket. Air-fry the chicken at 370°F for 20 minutes, flipping the pieces over halfway through the cooking process, taking care not to knock off the breading. Transfer the chicken to a plate, but do not cover. Repeat with the second batch of chicken.

5. Lower the temperature on the air fryer to 340°F. Flip the chicken back over and place the first batch of chicken on top of the second batch already in the basket. Air-fry for another 7 minutes and serve warm.

Appetizers And Snacks

Country Wings

Servings: 4
Cooking Time: 19 Minutes
Ingredients:

- 2 pounds chicken wings
- Marinade
- 1 cup buttermilk
- ½ teaspoon black pepper
- ½ teaspoon salt
- Coating
- 1 cup flour
- 1 cup panko breadcrumbs
- 2 teaspoons salt
- 2 tablespoons poultry seasoning
- oil for misting or cooking spray

Directions:

1. Cut the tips off the wings. Discard or freeze for stock. Cut remaining wing sections apart at the joint to make 2 pieces per wing. Place wings in a large bowl or plastic bag.
2. Mix together all marinade ingredients and pour over wings. Refrigerate for at least 1 hour but for no more than 8 hours.
3. Preheat air fryer to 360°F.
4. Mix all coating ingredients together in a shallow dish or on wax paper.
5. Remove wings from marinade, shaking off excess, and roll in coating mixture.
6. Spray both sides of each wing with oil or cooking spray.
7. Place wings in air fryer basket in single layer, close but not too crowded. Cook for 19minutes or until chicken is done and juices run clear.
8. Repeat step 7 to cook remaining wings.

Crispy Wontons

Servings: 8
Cooking Time: 10 Minutes
Ingredients:

- ½ cup refried beans
- 3 tablespoons salsa
- ¼ cup canned artichoke hearts, drained and patted dry
- ¼ cup frozen spinach, defrosted and squeezed dry
- 2 ounces cream cheese
- 1½ teaspoons dried oregano, divided
- ¼ teaspoon garlic powder
- ¼ teaspoon onion powder
- ½ teaspoon salt
- ¼ cup chopped pepperoni
- ¼ cup grated mozzarella cheese
- 1 tablespoon grated Parmesan
- 2 ounces cream cheese
- ½ teaspoon dried oregano
- 32 wontons
- 1 cup water

Directions:

1. Preheat the air fryer to 370°F.
2. In a medium bowl, mix together the refried beans and salsa.
3. In a second medium bowl, mix together the artichoke hearts, spinach, cream cheese, oregano, garlic powder, onion powder, and salt.
4. In a third medium bowl, mix together the pepperoni, mozzarella cheese, Parmesan cheese, cream cheese, and the remaining ½ teaspoon of oregano.
5. Get a towel lightly damp with water and ring it out. While working with the wontons, leave the

unfilled wontons under the damp towel so they don't dry out.

6. Working with 8 wontons at a time, place 2 teaspoons of one of the fillings into the center of the wonton, rotating among the different fillings (one filling per wonton). Working one at a time, use a pastry brush, dip the pastry brush into the water, and brush the edges of the dough with the water. Fold the dough in half to form a triangle and set aside. Continue until 8 wontons are formed. Spray the wontons with cooking spray and cover with a dry towel. Repeat until all 32 wontons have been filled.

7. Place the wontons into the air fryer basket, leaving space between the wontons, and cook for 5 minutes. Turn over and check for brownness, and then cook for another 5 minutes.

Warm And Salty Edamame

Servings: 4
Cooking Time: 10 Minutes
Ingredients:
- 1 pound Unshelled edamame
- Vegetable oil spray
- ¾ teaspoon Coarse sea salt or kosher salt

Directions:
1. Preheat the air fryer to 400°F.
2. Place the edamame in a large bowl and lightly coat them with vegetable oil spray. Toss well, spray again, and toss until they are evenly coated.
3. When the machine is at temperature, pour the edamame into the basket and air-fry, tossing the basket quite often to rearrange the edamame, for 7 minutes, or until warm and aromatic. (Air-fry for 10 minutes if the edamame were frozen and not thawed.)
4. Pour the edamame into a bowl and sprinkle the salt on top. Toss well, then set aside for a couple of minutes before serving with an empty bowl on the side for the pods.

Smoked Whitefish Spread

Servings: 1
Cooking Time: 10 Minutes
Ingredients:
- ¾ pound Boneless skinless white-flesh fish fillets, such as hake or trout
- 3 tablespoons Liquid smoke
- 3 tablespoons Regular, low-fat, or fat-free mayonnaise (gluten-free, if a concern)
- 2 teaspoons Jarred prepared white horseradish (optional)
- ¼ teaspoon Onion powder
- ¼ teaspoon Celery seeds
- ¼ teaspoon Table salt
- ¼ teaspoon Ground black pepper

Directions:
1. Put the fish fillets in a zip-closed bag, add the liquid smoke, and seal closed. Rub the liquid smoke all over the fish , then refrigerate the sealed bag for 2 hours.
2. Preheat the air fryer to 400°F.
3. Set a 12-inch piece of aluminum foil on your work surface. Remove the fish fillets from the bag and set them in the center of this piece of foil (the fillets can overlap). Fold the long sides of the foil together and crimp them closed. Make a tight seam so no steam can escape. Fold up the ends and crimp to seal well.
4. Set the packet in the basket and air-fry undisturbed for 10 minutes.
5. Use kitchen tongs to transfer the foil packet to a wire rack. Cool for a minute or so. Open the packet, transfer the fish to a plate, and refrigerate for 30 minutes.

6. Put the cold fish in a food processor. Add the mayonnaise, horseradish (if using), onion powder, celery seeds, salt, and pepper. Cover and pulse to a slightly coarse spread, certainly not fully smooth.

7. For a more traditional texture, put the fish fillets in a bowl, add the other ingredients, and stir with a wooden spoon, mashing the fish with everything else to make a coarse paste.

8. Scrape the spread into a bowl and serve at once, or cover with plastic wrap and store in the fridge for up to 4 days.

Asian Five-spice Wings

Servings: 4

Cooking Time: 15 Minutes

Ingredients:

- 2 pounds chicken wings
- ½ cup Asian-style salad dressing
- 2 tablespoons Chinese five-spice powder

Directions:

1. Cut off wing tips and discard or freeze for stock. Cut remaining wing pieces in two at the joint.

2. Place wing pieces in a large sealable plastic bag. Pour in the Asian dressing, seal bag, and massage the marinade into the wings until well coated. Refrigerate for at least an hour.

3. Remove wings from bag, drain off excess marinade, and place wings in air fryer basket.

4. Cook at 360°F for 15minutes or until juices run clear. About halfway through cooking time, shake the basket or stir wings for more even cooking.

5. Transfer cooked wings to plate in a single layer. Sprinkle half of the Chinese five-spice powder on the wings, turn, and sprinkle other side with remaining seasoning.

Greek Street Tacos

Servings: 8

Cooking Time: 3 Minutes

Ingredients:

- 8 small flour tortillas (4-inch diameter)
- 8 tablespoons hummus
- 4 tablespoons crumbled feta cheese
- 4 tablespoons chopped kalamata or other olives (optional)
- olive oil for misting

Directions:

1. Place 1 tablespoon of hummus or tapenade in the center of each tortilla. Top with 1 teaspoon of feta crumbles and 1 teaspoon of chopped olives, if using.

2. Using your finger or a small spoon, moisten the edges of the tortilla all around with water.

3. Fold tortilla over to make a half-moon shape. Press center gently. Then press the edges firmly to seal in the filling.

4. Mist both sides with olive oil.

5. Place in air fryer basket very close but try not to overlap.

6. Cook at 390°F for 3minutes, just until lightly browned and crispy.

Zucchini Fries With Roasted Garlic Aïoli

Servings: 4

Cooking Time: 12 Minutes

Ingredients:

- Roasted Garlic Aïoli:
- 1 teaspoon roasted garlic
- ½ cup mayonnaise
- 2 tablespoons olive oil
- juice of ½ lemon
- salt and pepper

- Zucchini Fries:
- ½ cup flour
- 2 eggs, beaten
- 1 cup seasoned breadcrumbs
- salt and pepper
- 1 large zucchini, cut into ½-inch sticks
- olive oil in a spray bottle, can or mister

Directions:

1. To make the aïoli, combine the roasted garlic, mayonnaise, olive oil and lemon juice in a bowl and whisk well. Season the aïoli with salt and pepper to taste.

2. Prepare the zucchini fries. Create a dredging station with three shallow dishes. Place the flour in the first shallow dish and season well with salt and freshly ground black pepper. Put the beaten eggs in the second shallow dish. In the third shallow dish, combine the breadcrumbs, salt and pepper. Dredge the zucchini sticks, coating with flour first, then dipping them into the eggs to coat, and finally tossing in breadcrumbs. Shake the dish with the breadcrumbs and pat the crumbs onto the zucchini sticks gently with your hands so they stick evenly.

3. Place the zucchini fries on a flat surface and let them sit at least 10 minutes before air-frying to let them dry out a little. Preheat the air fryer to 400°F.

4. Spray the zucchini sticks with olive oil, and place them into the air fryer basket. You can air-fry the zucchini in two layers, placing the second layer in the opposite direction to the first. Air-fry for 12 minutes turning and rotating the fries halfway through the cooking time. Spray with additional oil when you turn them over.

5. Serve zucchini fries warm with the roasted garlic aïoli.

Fried Brie With Cherry Tomatoes

Servings: 8

Cooking Time: 15 Minutes

Ingredients:

- 1 baguette*
- 2 pints red and yellow cherry tomatoes
- 1 tablespoon olive oil
- salt and freshly ground black pepper
- 1 teaspoon balsamic vinegar
- 1 tablespoon chopped fresh parsley
- 1 (8-ounce) wheel of Brie cheese
- olive oil
- ½ teaspoon Italian seasoning (optional)
- 1 tablespoon chopped fresh basil

Directions:

1. Preheat the air fryer to 350°F.

2. Start by making the crostini. Slice the baguette diagonally into ½-inch slices and brush the slices with olive oil on both sides. Air-fry the baguette slices at 350°F in batches for 6 minutes or until lightly browned on all sides. Set the bread aside on your serving platter.

3. Toss the cherry tomatoes in a bowl with the olive oil, salt and pepper. Air-fry the cherry tomatoes for 3 to 5 minutes, shaking the basket a few times during the cooking process. The tomatoes should be soft and some of them will burst open. Toss the warm tomatoes with the balsamic vinegar and fresh parsley and set aside.

4. Cut a circle of parchment paper the same size as your wheel of Brie cheese. Brush both sides of the Brie wheel with olive oil and sprinkle with Italian seasoning, if using. Place the circle of parchment paper on one side of the Brie and transfer the Brie to the air fryer basket, parchment side down. Air-fry at 350°F for 8 to

10 minutes, or until the Brie is slightly puffed and soft to the touch.

5. Watch carefully and remove the Brie before the rind cracks and the cheese starts to leak out. Transfer the wheel to your serving platter and top with the roasted tomatoes. Sprinkle with basil and serve with the toasted bread slices.

Zucchini Fritters

Servings: 8
Cooking Time: 10 Minutes
Ingredients:

- 2 cups grated zucchini
- ½ teaspoon sea salt
- 1 egg
- ½ teaspoon garlic powder
- ¼ teaspoon onion powder
- ¼ cup grated Parmesan cheese
- ½ cup all-purpose flour
- ¼ teaspoon baking powder
- ½ cup Greek yogurt or sour cream
- ½ lime, juiced
- ¼ cup chopped cilantro
- ¼ teaspoon ground cumin
- ¼ teaspoon salt

Directions:

1. Preheat the air fryer to 360°F.

2. In a large colander, place a kitchen towel. Inside the towel, place the grated zucchini and sprinkle the sea salt over the top. Let the zucchini sit for 5 minutes; then, using the towel, squeeze dry the zucchini.

3. In a medium bowl, mix together the egg, garlic powder, onion powder, Parmesan cheese, flour, and baking powder. Add in the grated zucchini, and stir until completely combined.

4. Pierce a piece of parchment paper with a fork 4 to 6 times. Place the parchment paper into the air fryer basket. Using a tablespoon, place 6 to 8 heaping tablespoons of fritter batter onto the parchment paper. Spray the fritters with cooking spray and cook for 5 minutes, turn the fritters over, and cook another 5 minutes.

5. Meanwhile, while the fritters are cooking, make the sauce. In a small bowl, whisk together the Greek yogurt or sour cream, lime juice, cilantro, cumin, and salt.

6. Repeat Steps 2–4 with the remaining batter.

Popcorn Chicken Bites

Servings: 2
Cooking Time: 8 Minutes
Ingredients:

- 1 pound chicken breasts, cutlets or tenders
- 1 cup buttermilk
- 3 to 6 dashes hot sauce (optional)
- 8 cups cornflakes (or 2 cups cornflake crumbs)
- ½ teaspoon salt
- 1 tablespoon butter, melted
- 2 tablespoons chopped fresh parsley

Directions:

1. Cut the chicken into bite-sized pieces (about 1-inch) and place them in a bowl with the buttermilk and hot sauce (if using). Cover and let the chicken marinate in the buttermilk for 1 to 3 hours in the refrigerator.

2. Preheat the air fryer to 380°F.

3. Crush the cornflakes into fine crumbs by either crushing them with your hands in a bowl, rolling them with a rolling pin in a plastic bag or processing them in a food processor. Place the crumbs in a bowl, add the salt, melted butter and parsley and mix well. Working in batches, remove the chicken from the buttermilk marinade, letting any excess drip off and transfer the chicken to the cornflakes. Toss the chicken pieces in the

cornflake mixture to coat evenly, pressing the crumbs onto the chicken.

4. Air-fry the chicken in two batches for 8 minutes per batch, shaking the basket halfway through the cooking process. Re-heat the first batch with the second batch for a couple of minutes if desired.

5. Serve the popcorn chicken bites warm with BBQ sauce or honey mustard for dipping.

Crab Toasts

Servings: 15
Cooking Time: 5 Minutes

Ingredients:
- 1 6-ounce can flaked crabmeat, well drained
- 3 tablespoons light mayonnaise
- ½ teaspoon lemon juice
- 1 teaspoon Worcestershire sauce
- ¼ cup shredded sharp Cheddar cheese
- ¼ cup shredded Parmesan cheese
- 1 loaf artisan bread, French bread, or baguette, cut into slices ⅜-inch thick

Directions:
1. Mix together all ingredients except the bread slices.
2. Spread each slice of bread with a thin layer of crabmeat mixture. (For a bread slice measuring 2 x 1½ inches you will need about ½ tablespoon of crab mixture.)
3. Place in air fryer basket in single layer and cook at 360°F for 5minutes or until tops brown and toast is crispy.
4. Repeat step 3 to cook remaining crab toasts.

Veggie Cheese Bites

Servings: 4
Cooking Time: 8 Minutes

Ingredients:
- 2 cups riced vegetables (see the Note below)
- ½ cup shredded zucchini
- ½ teaspoon garlic powder
- ¼ teaspoon black pepper
- ¼ teaspoon salt
- 1 large egg
- ¾ cup shredded cheddar cheese
- ⅓ cup whole-wheat flour

Directions:
1. Preheat the air fryer to 350°F.
2. In a large bowl, mix together the riced vegetables, zucchini, garlic powder, pepper, and salt. Mix in the egg. Stir in the shredded cheese and whole-wheat flour until a thick, doughlike consistency forms. If you need to, add 1 teaspoon of flour at a time so you can mold the batter into balls.
3. Using a 1-inch scoop, portion the batter out into about 12 balls.
4. Liberally spray the air fryer basket with olive oil spray. Then place the veggie bites inside. Leave enough room between each bite so the air can flow around them.
5. Cook for 8 minutes, or until the outside is slightly browned. Depending on the size of your air fryer, you may need to cook these in batches.
6. Remove and let cool slightly before serving.

Loaded Potato Skins

Servings: 8
Cooking Time: 8 Minutes

Ingredients:
- 12 round baby potatoes
- 3 ounces cream cheese
- 4 slices cooked bacon, crumbled or chopped
- 2 green onions, finely chopped
- ½ cup grated cheddar cheese, divided

- ¼ cup sour cream
- 1 tablespoon milk
- 2 teaspoons hot sauce

Directions:

1. Preheat the air fryer to 320°F.

2. Poke holes into the baby potatoes with a fork. Place the potatoes onto a microwave-safe plate and microwave on high for 4 to 5 minutes, or until soft to squeeze. Let the potatoes cool until they're safe to handle, about 5 minutes.

3. Meanwhile, in a medium bowl, mix together the cream cheese, bacon, green onions, and ¼ cup of the cheddar cheese; set aside.

4. Slice the baby potatoes in half. Using a spoon, scoop out the pulp, leaving enough pulp on the inside to retain the shape of the potato half. Place the potato pulp into the cream cheese mixture and mash together with a fork. Using a spoon, refill the potato halves with filling.

5. Place the potato halves into the air fryer basket and top with the remaining ¼ cup of cheddar cheese.

6. Cook the loaded baked potato bites in batches for 8 minutes.

7. Meanwhile, make the sour cream sauce. In a small bowl, whisk together the sour cream, milk, and hot sauce. Add more hot sauce if desired.

8. When the potatoes have all finished cooking, place them onto a serving platter and serve with sour cream sauce drizzled over the top or as a dip.

Spicy Sweet Potato Tater-tots

Servings: 6

Cooking Time: 10 Minutes

Ingredients:

- 6 cups filtered water
- 2 medium sweet potatoes, peeled and cut in half
- 1 teaspoon garlic powder
- ½ teaspoon black pepper, divided
- ½ teaspoon salt, divided
- 1 cup panko breadcrumbs
- 1 teaspoon blackened seasoning

Directions:

1. In a large stovetop pot, bring the water to a boil. Add the sweet potatoes and let boil about 10 minutes, until a metal fork prong can be inserted but the potatoes still have a slight give (not completely mashed).

2. Carefully remove the potatoes from the pot and let cool.

3. When you're able to touch them, grate the potatoes into a large bowl. Mix the garlic powder, ¼ teaspoon of the black pepper, and ¼ teaspoon of the salt into the potatoes. Place the mixture in the refrigerator and let set at least 45 minutes (if you're leaving them longer than 45 minutes, cover the bowl).

4. Before assembling, mix the breadcrumbs and blackened seasoning in a small bowl.

5. Remove the sweet potatoes from the refrigerator and preheat the air fryer to 400°F.

6. Assemble the tater-tots by using a teaspoon to portion batter evenly and form into a tater-tot shape. Roll each tater-tot in the breadcrumb mixture. Then carefully place the tater-tots in the air fryer basket. Be sure that you've liberally sprayed the air fryer basket with an olive oil mist. Repeat until tater-tots fill the basket without touching one another. You'll need to do multiple batches, depending on the size of your air fryer.

7. Cook the tater-tots for 3 to 6 minutes, flip, and cook another 3 to 6 minutes.

8. Remove from the air fryer carefully and keep warm until ready to serve.

Classic Chicken Wings

Servings: 8
Cooking Time: 20 Minutes
Ingredients:
- 16 chicken wings
- ¼ cup all-purpose flour
- ¼ teaspoon garlic powder
- ¼ teaspoon paprika
- ½ teaspoon salt
- ½ teaspoon black pepper
- ¼ cup butter
- ½ cup hot sauce
- ½ teaspoon Worcestershire sauce
- 2 ounces crumbled blue cheese, for garnish

Directions:
1. Preheat the air fryer to 380°F.
2. Pat the chicken wings dry with paper towels.
3. In a medium bowl, mix together the flour, garlic powder, paprika, salt, and pepper. Toss the chicken wings with the flour mixture, dusting off any excess.
4. Place the chicken wings in the air fryer basket, making sure that the chicken wings aren't touching. Cook the chicken wings for 10 minutes, turn over, and cook another 5 minutes. Raise the temperature to 400°F and continue crisping the chicken wings for an additional 3 to 5 minutes.
5. Meanwhile, in a microwave-safe bowl, melt the butter and hot sauce for 1 to 2 minutes in the microwave. Remove from the microwave and stir in the Worcestershire sauce.
6. When the chicken wings have cooked, immediately transfer the chicken wings into the hot sauce mixture. Serve the coated chicken wings on a plate, and top with crumbled blue cheese.

Fried Mozzarella Sticks

Servings: 7
Cooking Time: 5 Minutes

Ingredients:
- 7 1-ounce string cheese sticks, unwrapped
- ½ cup All-purpose flour or tapioca flour
- 2 Large egg(s), well beaten
- 2¼ cups Seasoned Italian-style dried bread crumbs (gluten-free, if a concern)
- Olive oil spray

Directions:
1. Unwrap the string cheese and place the pieces in the freezer for 20 minutes (but not longer, or they will be too frozen to soften in the time given in the air fryer).
2. Preheat the air fryer to 400°F.
3. Set up and fill three shallow soup plates or small pie plates on your counter: one for the flour, one for the egg(s), and one for the bread crumbs.
4. Dip a piece of cold string cheese in the flour until well coated (keep the others in the freezer). Gently tap off any excess flour, then set the stick in the egg(s). Roll it around to coat, let any excess egg mixture slip back into the rest, and set the stick in the bread crumbs. Gently roll it around to coat it evenly, even the ends. Now dip it back in the egg(s), then again in the bread crumbs, rolling it to coat well and evenly. Set the stick aside on a cutting board and coat the remaining pieces of string cheese in the same way.
5. Lightly coat the sticks all over with olive oil spray. Place them in the basket in one layer and air-fry undisturbed for 5 minutes, or until golden brown and crisp.
6. Remove the basket from the machine and cool for 5 minutes. Use a nonstick-safe spatula to transfer the mozzarella sticks to a serving platter. Serve hot.

Eggplant Fries

Servings: 4

Cooking Time: 8 Minutes

Ingredients:

- 1 medium eggplant
- 1 teaspoon ground coriander
- 1 teaspoon cumin
- 1 teaspoon garlic powder
- ½ teaspoon salt
- 1 cup crushed panko breadcrumbs
- 1 large egg
- 2 tablespoons water
- oil for misting or cooking spray

Directions:

1. Peel and cut the eggplant into fat fries, ⅜- to ½-inch thick.

2. Preheat air fryer to 390°F.

3. In a small cup, mix together the coriander, cumin, garlic, and salt.

4. Combine 1 teaspoon of the seasoning mix and panko crumbs in a shallow dish.

5. Place eggplant fries in a large bowl, sprinkle with remaining seasoning, and stir well to combine.

6. Beat eggs and water together and pour over eggplant fries. Stir to coat.

7. Remove eggplant from egg wash, shaking off excess, and roll in panko crumbs.

8. Spray with oil.

9. Place half of the fries in air fryer basket. You should have only a single layer, but it's fine if they overlap a little.

10. Cook for 5minutes. Shake basket, mist lightly with oil, and cook 3 minutes longer, until browned and crispy.

11. Repeat step 10 to cook remaining eggplant.

Scotch Eggs

Servings: 6

Cooking Time: 12 Minutes

Ingredients:

- 7 Large eggs
- 1½ cups Corn flake crumbs (gluten-free, if a concern)
- 1½ pounds Bulk mild or hot breakfast sausage meat (gluten-free, if a concern)
- Vegetable oil spray
- For garnishing Coarse sea salt or kosher salt

Directions:

1. Bring a little more than 1 inch of water to a boil in a large saucepan set over high heat. Meanwhile, prepare a big bowl of ice water.

2. Set 4, 6, or 8 of the eggs in a vegetable steamer basket and lower them into the pot. Cover, reduce the heat to low, and steam for 10 minutes. Drain the eggs into a colander set in the sink, then put them in the ice water. Cool for 10 minutes, then peel the eggs. (Be careful: the whites are set but not the yolks!)

3. Preheat the air fryer to 375°F (or 380°F or 390°F, if one of these is the closest setting).

4. Lay a sheet of plastic wrap on a clean, dry work surface. Place ¼ pound (4 ounces) of the sausage meat in the center of the sheet, then press the sausage into an oval 7 inches long and about 5 inches wide at its widest part. Place a peeled egg in the center of the sausage, then carefully and gently (no awards for speed!) use the plastic wrap to fold the sausage up and around the egg. Remove the plastic wrap, dampen your clean hands, then smooth and seal the sausage over the egg. Repeat with the remaining sausage and eggs, using a fresh sheet of plastic wrap each time.

5. Set up and fill two shallow soup plates or small pie plates on your counter: one with the remaining egg(s) in it, well beaten until uniform, and the other with the corn flake crumbs. Roll the sausage-covered egg in the beaten egg. Let the excess slip back into the rest, then set the coated egg in the corn flake crumbs. Roll the egg in the corn flake crumbs to coat it evenly and well, even on the ends. Set aside, then coat the remaining sausage-covered eggs.

6. Give the crumbed eggs a generous coating of vegetable oil spray. Set them in the basket in one layer and air-fry undisturbed for 12 minutes, or until the coating is well browned. If the air fryer is at 390°F, the Scotch eggs may be done in 10 minutes.

7. Use kitchen tongs to transfer the eggs to a wire rack. Cool for at least 5 minutes or up to 30 minutes before serving. Split the eggs in half, sprinkle them with salt, and relish every bite.

Granola Three Ways

Servings: 4

Cooking Time: 10 Minutes

Ingredients:
- Nantucket Granola
- ¼ cup maple syrup
- ¼ cup dark brown sugar
- 1 tablespoon butter
- 1 teaspoon vanilla extract
- 1 cup rolled oats
- ½ cup dried cranberries
- ½ cup walnuts, chopped
- ¼ cup pumpkin seeds
- ¼ cup shredded coconut
- Blueberry Delight
- ¼ cup honey
- ¼ cup light brown sugar
- 1 tablespoon butter
- 1 teaspoon lemon extract
- 1 cup rolled oats
- ½ cup sliced almonds
- ½ cup dried blueberries
- ¼ cup pumpkin seeds
- ¼ cup sunflower seeds
- Cherry Black Forest Mix
- ¼ cup honey
- ¼ cup light brown sugar
- 1 tablespoon butter
- 1 teaspoon almond extract
- 1 cup rolled oats
- ½ cup sliced almonds
- ½ cup dried cherries
- ¼ cup shredded coconut
- ¼ cup dark chocolate chips
- oil for misting or cooking spray

Directions:
1. Combine the syrup or honey, brown sugar, and butter in a small saucepan or microwave-safe bowl. Heat and stir just until butter melts and sugar dissolves. Stir in the extract.

2. Place all other dry ingredients in a large bowl. (For the Cherry Black Forest Mix, don't add the chocolate chips yet.)

3. Pour melted butter mixture over dry ingredients and stir until oat mixture is well coated.

4. Lightly spray a baking pan with oil or cooking spray.

5. Pour granola into pan and cook at 390°F for 5minutes. Stir. Continue cooking for 5minutes, stirring every minute or two, until golden brown. Watch closely. Once the mixture begins to brown, it will cook quickly.

6. Remove granola from pan and spread on wax paper. It will become crispier as it cools.

7. For the Cherry Black Forest Mix, stir in chocolate chips after granola has cooled completely.

8. Store in an airtight container.

Baba Ghanouj

Servings: 2
Cooking Time: 40 Minutes
Ingredients:
- 2 Small (12-ounce) purple Italian eggplant(s)
- ¼ cup Olive oil
- ¼ cup Tahini
- ½ teaspoon Ground black pepper
- ¼ teaspoon Onion powder
- ¼ teaspoon Mild smoked paprika (optional)
- Up to 1 teaspoon Table salt

Directions:
1. Preheat the air fryer to 400°F.

2. Prick the eggplant(s) on all sides with a fork. When the machine is at temperature, set the eggplant(s) in the basket in one layer. Air-fry undisturbed for 40 minutes, or until blackened and soft.

3. Remove the basket from the machine. Cool the eggplant(s) in the basket for 20 minutes.

4. Use a nonstick-safe spatula, and perhaps a flatware tablespoon for balance, to gently transfer the eggplant(s) to a bowl. The juices will run out. Make sure the bowl is close to the basket. Split the eggplant(s) open.

5. Scrape the soft insides of half an eggplant into a food processor. Repeat with the remaining piece(s). Add any juices from the bowl to the eggplant in the food processor, but discard the skins and stems.

6. Add the olive oil, tahini, pepper, onion powder, and smoked paprika (if using). Add about half the salt, then cover and process until smooth, stopping the machine at least once to scrape down the inside of the canister. Check the spread for salt and add more as needed. Scrape the baba ghanouj into a bowl and serve warm, or set aside at room temperature for up to 2 hours, or cover and store in the refrigerator for up to 4 days.

Homemade Pretzel Bites

Servings: 8
Cooking Time: 6 Minutes
Ingredients:
- 4¾ cups filtered water, divided
- 1 tablespoon butter
- 1 package fast-rising yeast
- ½ teaspoon salt
- 2⅓ cups bread flour
- 2 tablespoons baking soda
- 2 egg whites
- 1 teaspoon kosher salt

Directions:
1. Preheat the air fryer to 370°F.

2. In a large microwave-safe bowl, add ¾ cup of the water. Heat for 40 seconds in the microwave. Remove and whisk in the butter; then mix in the yeast and salt. Let sit 5 minutes.

3. Using a stand mixer with a dough hook attachment, add the yeast liquid and mix in the bread flour ⅓ cup at a time until all the flour is added and a dough is formed.

4. Remove the bowl from the stand; then let the dough rise 1 hour in a warm space, covered with a kitchen towel.

5. After the dough has doubled in size, remove from the bowl and punch down a few times on a lightly floured flat surface.

6. Divide the dough into 4 balls; then roll each ball out into a long, skinny, sticklike shape. Using a sharp knife, cut each dough stick into 6 pieces.

7. Repeat Step 6 for the remaining dough balls until you have about 24 bites formed.

8. Heat the remaining 4 cups of water over the stovetop in a medium pot with the baking soda stirred in.

9. Drop the pretzel bite dough into the hot water and let boil for 60 seconds, remove, and let slightly cool.

10. Lightly brush the top of each bite with the egg whites, and then cover with a pinch of kosher salt.

11. Spray the air fryer basket with olive oil spray and place the pretzel bites on top. Cook for 6 to 8 minutes, or until lightly browned. Remove and keep warm.

12. Repeat until all pretzel bites are cooked.

13. Serve warm.

Chicken Shawarma Bites

Servings: 6

Cooking Time: 22 Minutes

Ingredients:

- 1½ pounds Boneless skinless chicken thighs, trimmed of any fat and cut into 1-inch pieces
- 1½ tablespoons Olive oil
- Up to 1½ tablespoons Minced garlic
- ½ teaspoon Table salt
- ¼ teaspoon Ground cardamom
- ¼ teaspoon Ground cinnamon
- ¼ teaspoon Ground cumin
- ¼ teaspoon Mild paprika
- Up to a ¼ teaspoon Grated nutmeg
- ¼ teaspoon Ground black pepper

Directions:

1. Preheat the air fryer to 400°F.

2. Mix all the ingredients in a large bowl until the chicken is thoroughly and evenly coated in the oil and spices.

3. When the machine is at temperature, scrape the coated chicken pieces into the basket and spread them out into one layer as much as you can. Air-fry for 22 minutes, shaking the basket at least three times during cooking to rearrange the pieces, until well browned and crisp.

4. Pour the chicken pieces onto a wire rack. Cool for 5 minutes before serving.

Herbed Cheese Brittle

Servings: 4

Cooking Time: 5 Minutes

Ingredients:

- ½ cup shredded Parmesan cheese
- ½ cup shredded white cheddar cheese
- 1 tablespoon fresh chopped rosemary
- 1 teaspoon garlic powder
- 1 large egg white

Directions:

1. Preheat the air fryer to 400°F.

2. In a large bowl, mix the cheeses, rosemary, and garlic powder. Mix in the egg white. Then pour the batter into a 7-inch pan (or an air-fryer-compatible pan). Place the pan in the air fryer basket and cook for 4 to 5 minutes, or until the cheese is melted and slightly browned.

3. Remove the pan from the air fryer, and let it cool for 2 minutes. Invert the pan before the cheese brittle completely cools but is semi-hardened to allow it to easily slide out of the pan.

4. Let the pan cool another 5 minutes. Break into pieces and serve.

Spanakopita Spinach, Feta And Pine Nut Phyllo Bites

Servings: 8

Cooking Time: 10 Minutes

Ingredients:

- ½ (10-ounce) package frozen spinach, thawed and squeezed dry (about 1 cup)
- ¾ cup crumbled feta cheese
- ¼ cup grated Parmesan cheese
- ¼ cup pine nuts, toasted
- ⅛ teaspoon ground nutmeg
- 1 egg, lightly beaten
- ½ teaspoon salt
- freshly ground black pepper
- 6 sheets phyllo dough
- ½ cup butter, melted

Directions:

1. Combine the spinach, cheeses, pine nuts, nutmeg and egg in a bowl. Season with salt and freshly ground black pepper.

2. While building the phyllo triangles, always keep the dough sheets you are not working with covered with plastic wrap and a damp clean kitchen towel. Remove one sheet of the phyllo and place it on a flat surface. Brush the phyllo sheet with melted butter and then layer another sheet of phyllo on top. Brush the second sheet of phyllo with butter. Cut the layered phyllo sheets into 6 strips, about 2½- to 3-inches wide.

3. Place a heaping tablespoon of the spinach filling at the end of each strip of dough. Fold the bottom right corner of the strip over the filling towards the left edge of the strip to make a triangle. Continue to fold the phyllo dough around the spinach as you would fold a flag, making triangle after triangle. Brush the outside of the phyllo triangle with more melted butter and set it aside until you've finished the 6 strips of dough, making 6 triangles.

4. Preheat the air fryer to 350°F.

5. Transfer the first six phyllo triangles to the air fryer basket and air-fry for 5 minutes. Turn the triangles over and air-fry for another 5 minutes.

6. While the first batch of triangles is air-frying, build another set of triangles and air-fry in the same manner. You should do three batches total. These can be warmed in the air fryer for a minute or two just before serving if you like.

Cauliflower "tater" Tots

Servings: 6

Cooking Time: 10 Minutes

Ingredients:

- 1 head of cauliflower
- 2 eggs
- ¼ cup all-purpose flour*
- ½ cup grated Parmesan cheese
- 1 teaspoon salt
- freshly ground black pepper
- vegetable or olive oil, in a spray bottle

Directions:

1. Grate the head of cauliflower with a box grater or finely chop it in a food processor. You should have about 3½ cups. Place the chopped cauliflower in the center of a clean kitchen towel and twist the towel tightly to squeeze all the water out of the cauliflower. (This can be done in two batches to make it easier to drain all the water from the cauliflower.)

2. Place the squeezed cauliflower in a large bowl. Add the eggs, flour, Parmesan cheese, salt and freshly ground black pepper. Shape the cauliflower into small cylinders or "tater tot" shapes, rolling roughly one tablespoon of the mixture at a time. Place the tots on a cookie sheet

lined with paper towel to absorb any residual moisture. Spray the cauliflower tots all over with oil.

3. Preheat the air fryer to 400°F.

4. Air-fry the tots at 400°F, one layer at a time for 10 minutes, turning them over for the last few minutes of the cooking process for even browning. Season with salt and black pepper. Serve hot with your favorite dipping sauce.

Beet Chips

Servings: 4

Cooking Time: 20 Minutes

Ingredients:

- 2 large red beets, washed and skinned
- 1 tablespoon avocado oil
- ¼ teaspoon salt

Directions:

1. Preheat the air fryer to 330°F.

2. Using a mandolin or sharp knife, slice the beets in ⅛-inch slices. Place them in a bowl of water and let them soak for 30 minutes. Drain the water and pat the beets dry with a paper towel or kitchen cloth.

3. In a medium bowl, toss the beets with avocado oil and sprinkle them with salt.

4. Lightly spray the air fryer basket with olive oil mist and place the beet chips into the basket. To allow for even cooking, don't overlap the beets; cook in batches if necessary.

5. Cook the beet chips 15 to 20 minutes, shaking the basket every 5 minutes, until the outer edges of the beets begin to flip up like a chip. Remove from the basket and serve warm. Repeat with the remaining chips until they're all cooked.

Carrot Chips

Servings: 4

Cooking Time: 10 Minutes

Ingredients:

- 1 pound carrots, thinly sliced
- 2 tablespoons extra-virgin olive oil
- ¼ teaspoon garlic powder
- ¼ teaspoon black pepper
- ½ teaspoon salt

Directions:

1. Preheat the air fryer to 390°F.

2. In a medium bowl, toss the carrot slices with the olive oil, garlic powder, pepper, and salt.

3. Liberally spray the air fryer basket with olive oil mist.

4. Place the carrot slices in the air fryer basket. To allow for even cooking, don't overlap the carrots; cook in batches if necessary.

5. Cook for 5 minutes, shake the basket, and cook another 5 minutes.

6. Remove from the basket and serve warm. Repeat with the remaining carrot slices until they're all cooked.

Cinnamon Apple Crisps

Servings: 1

Cooking Time: 22 Minutes

Ingredients:

- 1 large apple
- ½ teaspoon ground cinnamon
- 2 teaspoons avocado oil or coconut oil

Directions:

1. Preheat the air fryer to 300°F.

2. Using a mandolin or knife, slice the apples to ¼-inch thickness. Pat the apples dry with a paper towel or kitchen cloth. Sprinkle the apple slices

with ground cinnamon. Spray or drizzle the oil over the top of the apple slices and toss to coat.

3. Place the apple slices in the air fryer basket. To allow for even cooking, don't overlap the slices; cook in batches if necessary.

4. Cook for 20 minutes, shaking the basket every 5 minutes. After 20 minutes, increase the air fryer temperature to 330°F and cook another 2 minutes, shaking the basket every 30 seconds. Remove the apples from the basket before they get too dark.

5. Spread the chips out onto paper towels to cool completely, at least 5 minutes. Repeat with the remaining apple slices until they're all cooked.

Bacon Candy

Servings: 6

Cooking Time: 6 Minutes

Ingredients:

- 1½ tablespoons Honey
- 1 teaspoon White wine vinegar
- 3 Extra thick–cut bacon strips, halved widthwise (gluten-free, if a concern)
- ½ teaspoon Ground black pepper

Directions:

1. Preheat the air fryer to 350°F .

2. Whisk the honey and vinegar in a small bowl until incorporated.

3. When the machine is at temperature, remove the basket. Lay the bacon strip halves in the basket in one layer. Brush the tops with the honey mixture; sprinkle each bacon strip evenly with black pepper.

4. Return the basket to the machine and air-fry undisturbed for 6 minutes, or until the bacon is crunchy. Or a little less time if you prefer bacon that's still pliable, an extra minute if you want the bacon super crunchy. Take care that the honey coating doesn't burn. Remove the basket from the machine and set aside for 5 minutes. Use kitchen tongs to transfer the bacon strips to a serving plate.

Fried Goat Cheese

Servings: 3

Cooking Time: 4 Minutes

Ingredients:

- 7 ounces 1- to 1½-inch-diameter goat cheese log
- 2 Large egg(s)
- 1¾ cups Plain dried bread crumbs (gluten-free, if a concern)
- Vegetable oil spray

Directions:

1. Slice the goat cheese log into ½-inch-thick rounds. Set these flat on a small cutting board, a small baking sheet, or a large plate. Freeze uncovered for 30 minutes.

2. Preheat the air fryer to 400°F.

3. Set up and fill two shallow soup plates or small pie plates on your counter: one in which you whisk the egg(s) until uniform and the other for the bread crumbs.

4. Take the goat cheese rounds out of the freezer. With clean, dry hands, dip one round in the egg(s) to coat it on all sides. Let the excess egg slip back into the rest, then dredge the round in the bread crumbs, turning it to coat all sides, even the edges. Repeat this process—egg, then bread crumbs—

for a second coating. Coat both sides of the round and its edges with vegetable oil spray, then set it aside. Continue double-dipping, double-dredging, and spraying the remaining rounds.

5. Place the rounds in one layer in the basket. Air-fry undisturbed for 4 minutes, or until lightly browned and crunchy. Do not overcook. Some of the goat cheese may break through the crust. A few little breaks are fine but stop the cooking before the coating reaches structural failure.

6. Remove the basket from the machine and set aside for 3 minutes. Use a nonstick-safe spatula, and maybe a flatware fork for balance, to transfer the rounds to a wire rack. Cool for 5 minutes more before serving.

Beef，Pork & Lamb Recipes

Venison Backstrap

Servings: 4
Cooking Time: 10 Minutes
Ingredients:
- 2 eggs
- ¼ cup milk
- 1 cup whole wheat flour
- ½ teaspoon salt
- ¼ teaspoon pepper
- 1 pound venison backstrap, sliced
- salt and pepper
- oil for misting or cooking spray

Directions:
1. Beat together eggs and milk in a shallow dish.
2. In another shallow dish, combine the flour, salt, and pepper. Stir to mix well.
3. Sprinkle venison steaks with additional salt and pepper to taste. Dip in flour, egg wash, then in flour again, pressing in coating.
4. Spray steaks with oil or cooking spray on both sides.
5. Cooking in 2 batches, place steaks in the air fryer basket in a single layer. Cook at 360°F for 8minutes. Spray with oil, turn over, and spray other side. Cook for 2 minutes longer, until coating is crispy brown and meat is done to your liking.
6. Repeat to cook remaining venison.

Lamb Burger With Feta And Olives

Servings: 3
Cooking Time: 16 Minutes
Ingredients:
- 2 teaspoons olive oil
- ⅓ onion, finely chopped
- 1 clove garlic, minced
- 1 pound ground lamb
- 2 tablespoons fresh parsley, finely chopped
- 1½ teaspoons fresh oregano, finely chopped
- ½ cup black olives, finely chopped
- ⅓ cup crumbled feta cheese
- ½ teaspoon salt
- freshly ground black pepper
- 4 thick pita breads
- toppings and condiments

Directions:
1. Preheat a medium skillet over medium-high heat on the stovetop. Add the olive oil and cook the onion until tender, but not browned – about 4 to 5 minutes. Add the garlic and cook for another minute. Transfer the onion and garlic to a mixing bowl and add the ground lamb, parsley, oregano, olives, feta cheese, salt and pepper. Gently mix the ingredients together.
2. Divide the mixture into 3 or 4 equal portions and then form the hamburgers, being careful not to over-handle the meat. One good way to do this is to throw the meat back and forth between your hands like a baseball, packing the meat each time you catch it. Flatten the balls into patties, making an indentation in the center of each patty. Flatten the sides of the patties as well to make it easier to fit them into the air fryer basket.
3. Preheat the air fryer to 370°F.
4. If you don't have room for all four burgers, air-fry two or three burgers at a time for 8 minutes at 370°F. Flip the burgers over and air-fry for another 8 minutes. If you cooked your burgers in batches, return the first batch of burgers to the air fryer for the last two minutes of cooking to re-heat. This should give you a

medium-well burger. If you'd prefer a medium-rare burger, shorten the cooking time to about 13 minutes. Remove the burgers to a resting plate and let the burgers rest for a few minutes before dressing and serving.

5. While the burgers are resting, toast the pita breads in the air fryer for 2 minutes. Tuck the burgers into the toasted pita breads, or wrap the pitas around the burgers and serve with a tzatziki sauce or some mayonnaise.

Crispy Pork Medallions With Radicchio And Endive Salad

Servings: 4

Cooking Time: 7 Minutes

Ingredients:

- 1 (8-ounce) pork tenderloin
- salt and freshly ground black pepper
- ¼ cup flour
- 2 eggs, lightly beaten
- ¾ cup cracker meal
- 1 teaspoon paprika
- 1 teaspoon dry mustard
- 1 teaspoon garlic powder
- 1 teaspoon dried thyme
- 1 teaspoon salt
- vegetable or canola oil, in spray bottle
- Vinaigrette
- ¼ cup white balsamic vinegar
- 2 tablespoons agave syrup (or honey or maple syrup)
- 1 tablespoon Dijon mustard
- juice of ½ lemon
- 2 tablespoons chopped chervil or flat-leaf parsley
- salt and freshly ground black pepper
- ½ cup extra-virgin olive oil

- Radicchio and Endive Salad
- 1 heart romaine lettuce, torn into large pieces
- ½ head radicchio, coarsely chopped
- 2 heads endive, sliced
- ½ cup cherry tomatoes, halved
- 3 ounces fresh mozzarella, diced
- salt and freshly ground black pepper

Directions:

1. Slice the pork tenderloin into 1-inch slices. Using a meat pounder, pound the pork slices into thin ½-inch medallions. Generously season the pork with salt and freshly ground black pepper on both sides.

2. Set up a dredging station using three shallow dishes. Place the flour in one dish and the beaten eggs in a second dish. Combine the cracker meal, paprika, dry mustard, garlic powder, thyme and salt in a third dish.

3. Preheat the air fryer to 400°F.

4. Dredge the pork medallions in flour first and then into the beaten egg. Let the excess egg drip off and coat both sides of the medallions with the cracker meal crumb mixture. Spray both sides of the coated medallions with vegetable or canola oil.

5. Air-fry the medallions in two batches at 400°F for 5 minutes. Once you have air-fried all the medallions, flip them all over and return the first batch of medallions back into the air fryer on top of the second batch. Air-fry at 400°F for an additional 2 minutes.

6. While the medallions are cooking, make the salad and dressing. Whisk the white balsamic vinegar, agave syrup, Dijon mustard, lemon juice, chervil, salt and pepper together in a small bowl. Whisk in the olive oil slowly until combined and thickened.

7. Combine the romaine lettuce, radicchio, endive, cherry tomatoes, and mozzarella cheese in

a large salad bowl. Drizzle the dressing over the vegetables and toss to combine. Season with salt and freshly ground black pepper.

8. Serve the pork medallions warm on or beside the salad.

Perfect Pork Chops

Servings: 3
Cooking Time: 10 Minutes
Ingredients:
- ¾ teaspoon Mild paprika
- ¾ teaspoon Dried thyme
- ¾ teaspoon Onion powder
- ¼ teaspoon Garlic powder
- ¼ teaspoon Table salt
- ¼ teaspoon Ground black pepper
- 3 6-ounce boneless center-cut pork loin chops
- Vegetable oil spray

Directions:
1. Preheat the air fryer to 400°F.
2. Mix the paprika, thyme, onion powder, garlic powder, salt, and pepper in a small bowl until well combined. Massage this mixture into both sides of the chops. Generously coat both sides of the chops with vegetable oil spray.
3. When the machine is at temperature, set the chops in the basket with as much air space between them as possible. Air-fry undisturbed for 10 minutes, or until an instant-read meat thermometer inserted into the thickest part of a chop registers 145°F.
4. Use kitchen tongs to transfer the chops to a cutting board or serving plates. Cool for 5 minutes before serving.

Pork Taco Gorditas

Servings: 4

Cooking Time: 21 Minutes
Ingredients:
- 1 pound lean ground pork
- 2 tablespoons chili powder
- 2 tablespoons ground cumin
- 1 teaspoon dried oregano
- 2 teaspoons paprika
- 1 teaspoon garlic powder
- ½ cup water
- 1 (15-ounce) can pinto beans, drained and rinsed
- ½ cup taco sauce
- salt and freshly ground black pepper
- 2 cups grated Cheddar cheese
- 5 (12-inch) flour tortillas
- 4 (8-inch) crispy corn tortilla shells
- 4 cups shredded lettuce
- 1 tomato, diced
- ⅓ cup sliced black olives
- sour cream, for serving
- tomato salsa, for serving

Directions:
1. Preheat the air fryer to 400°F.
2. Place the ground pork in the air fryer basket and air-fry at 400°F for 10 minutes, stirring a few times during the cooking process to gently break up the meat. Combine the chili powder, cumin, oregano, paprika, garlic powder and water in a small bowl. Stir the spice mixture into the browned pork. Stir in the beans and taco sauce and air-fry for an additional minute. Transfer the pork mixture to a bowl. Season to taste with salt and freshly ground black pepper.
3. Sprinkle ½ cup of the shredded cheese in the center of four of the flour tortillas, making sure to leave a 2-inch border around the edge free of cheese and filling. Divide the pork mixture among the four tortillas, placing it on top of the

cheese. Place a crunchy corn tortilla on top of the pork and top with shredded lettuce, diced tomatoes, and black olives. Cut the remaining flour tortilla into 4 quarters. These quarters of tortilla will serve as the bottom of the gordita. Place one quarter tortilla on top of each gordita and fold the edges of the bottom flour tortilla up over the sides, enclosing the filling. While holding the seams down, brush the bottom of the gordita with olive oil and place the seam side down on the countertop while you finish the remaining three gorditas.

4. Preheat the air fryer to 380°F.

5. Air-fry one gordita at a time. Transfer the gordita carefully to the air fryer basket, seam side down. Brush or spray the top tortilla with oil and air-fry for 5 minutes. Carefully turn the gordita over and air-fry for an additional 5 minutes, until both sides are browned. When finished air frying all four gorditas, layer them back into the air fryer for an additional minute to make sure they are all warm before serving with sour cream and salsa.

Brie And Cranberry Burgers

Servings: 3
Cooking Time: 9 Minutes
Ingredients:
- 1 pound ground beef (80% lean)
- 1 tablespoon chopped fresh thyme
- 1 tablespoon Worcestershire sauce
- ½ teaspoon salt
- freshly ground black pepper
- 1 (4-ounce) wheel of Brie cheese, sliced
- handful of arugula
- 3 or 4 brioche hamburger buns (or potato hamburger buns), toasted
- ¼ to ½ cup whole berry cranberry sauce
Directions:

1. Combine the beef, thyme, Worcestershire sauce, salt and pepper together in a large bowl and mix well. Divide the meat into 4 (¼-pound) portions or 3 larger portions and then form them into burger patties, being careful not to over-handle the meat.

2. Preheat the air fryer to 390°F and pour a little water into the bottom of the air fryer drawer. (This will help prevent the grease that drips into the bottom drawer from burning and smoking.)

3. Transfer the burgers to the air fryer basket. Air-fry the burgers at 390°F for 5 minutes. Flip the burgers over and air-fry for another 2 minutes. Top each burger with a couple slices of brie and air-fry for another minute or two, just to soften the cheese.

4. Build the burgers by placing a few leaves of arugula on the bottom bun, adding the burger and a spoonful of cranberry sauce on top. Top with the other half of the hamburger bun and enjoy.

Vietnamese Shaking Beef

Servings: 3
Cooking Time: 7 Minutes
Ingredients:
- 1 pound Beef tenderloin, cut into 1-inch cubes
- 1 tablespoon Regular or low-sodium soy sauce or gluten-free tamari sauce
- 1 tablespoon Fish sauce (gluten-free, if a concern)
- 1 tablespoon Dark brown sugar
- 1½ teaspoons Ground black pepper
- 3 Medium scallions, trimmed and thinly sliced
- 2 tablespoons Butter
- 1½ teaspoons Minced garlic

Directions:

1. Mix the beef, soy or tamari sauce, fish sauce, and brown sugar in a bowl until well combined. Cover and refrigerate for at least 2 hours or up to 8 hours, tossing the beef at least twice in the marinade.

2. Put a 6-inch round or square cake pan in an air-fryer basket for a small batch, a 7-inch round or square cake pan for a medium batch, or an 8-inch round or square cake pan for a large one. Or put one of these on the rack of a toaster oven–style air fryer. Heat the machine with the pan in it to 400°F. When the machine it at temperature, let the pan sit in the heat for 2 to 3 minutes so that it gets very hot.

3. Use a slotted spoon to transfer the beef to the pan, leaving any marinade behind in the bowl. Spread the meat into as close to an even layer as you can. Air-fry undisturbed for 5 minutes. Meanwhile, discard the marinade, if any.

4. Add the scallions, butter, and garlic to the beef. Air-fry for 2 minutes, tossing and rearranging the beef and scallions repeatedly, perhaps every 20 seconds.

5. Remove the basket from the machine and let the meat cool in the pan for a couple of minutes before serving.

Bourbon Bacon Burgers

Servings: 2
Cooking Time: 23-28 Minutes

Ingredients:

- 1 tablespoon bourbon
- 2 tablespoons brown sugar
- 3 strips maple bacon, cut in half
- ¾ pound ground beef (80% lean)
- 1 tablespoon minced onion
- 2 tablespoons BBQ sauce
- ½ teaspoon salt
- freshly ground black pepper
- 2 slices Colby Jack cheese (or Monterey Jack)
- 2 Kaiser rolls
- lettuce and tomato, for serving
- Zesty Burger Sauce:
- 2 tablespoons BBQ sauce
- 2 tablespoons mayonnaise
- ¼ teaspoon ground paprika
- freshly ground black pepper

Directions:

1. Preheat the air fryer to 390°F and pour a little water into the bottom of the air fryer drawer. (This will help prevent the grease that drips into the bottom drawer from burning and smoking.)

2. Combine the bourbon and brown sugar in a small bowl. Place the bacon strips in the air fryer basket and brush with the brown sugar mixture. Air-fry at 390°F for 4 minutes. Flip the bacon over, brush with more brown sugar and air-fry at 390°F for an additional 4 minutes until crispy.

3. While the bacon is cooking, make the burger patties. Combine the ground beef, onion, BBQ sauce, salt and pepper in a large bowl. Mix together thoroughly with your hands and shape the meat into 2 patties.

4. Transfer the burger patties to the air fryer basket and air-fry the burgers at 370°F for 15 to 20 minutes, depending on how you like your burger cooked (15 minutes for rare to medium-rare; 20 minutes for well-done). Flip the burgers over halfway through the cooking process.

5. While the burgers are air-frying, make the burger sauce by combining the BBQ sauce, mayonnaise, paprika and freshly ground black pepper in a bowl.

6. When the burgers are cooked to your liking, top each patty with a slice of Colby Jack cheese

and air-fry for an additional minute, just to melt the cheese. (You might want to pin the cheese slice to the burger with a toothpick to prevent it from blowing off in your air fryer.) Spread the sauce on the inside of the Kaiser rolls, place the burgers on the rolls, top with the bourbon bacon, lettuce and tomato and enjoy!

Sausage-cheese Calzone

Servings: 8
Cooking Time: 8 Minutes

Ingredients:
- Crust
- 2 cups white wheat flour, plus more for kneading and rolling
- 1 package (¼ ounce) RapidRise yeast
- 1 teaspoon salt
- ½ teaspoon dried basil
- 1 cup warm water (115°F to 125°F)
- 2 teaspoons olive oil
- Filling
- ¼ pound Italian sausage
- ½ cup ricotta cheese
- 4 ounces mozzarella cheese, shredded
- ¼ cup grated Parmesan cheese
- oil for misting or cooking spray
- marinara sauce for serving

Directions:
1. Crumble Italian sausage into air fryer baking pan and cook at 390°F for 5minutes. Stir, breaking apart, and cook for 3 to 4minutes, until well done. Remove and set aside on paper towels to drain.
2. To make dough, combine flour, yeast, salt, and basil. Add warm water and oil and stir until a soft dough forms. Turn out onto lightly floured board and knead for 3 or 4minutes. Let dough rest for 10minutes.
3. To make filling, combine the three cheeses in a medium bowl and mix well. Stir in the cooked sausage.
4. Cut dough into 8 pieces.
5. Working with 4 pieces of the dough, press each into a circle about 5 inches in diameter. Top each dough circle with 2 heaping tablespoons of filling. Fold over to create a half-moon shape and press edges firmly together. Be sure that edges are firmly sealed to prevent leakage. Spray both sides with oil or cooking spray.
6. Place 4 calzones in air fryer basket and cook at 360°F for 5minutes. Mist with oil and cook for 3 minutes, until crust is done and nicely browned.
7. While the first batch is cooking, press out the remaining dough, fill, and shape into calzones.
8. Spray both sides with oil and cook for 5minutes. If needed, mist with oil and continue cooking for 3 minutes longer. This second batch will cook a little faster than the first because your air fryer is already hot.
9. Serve with marinara sauce on the side for dipping.

Spicy Hoisin Bbq Pork Chops

Servings: 2
Cooking Time: 12 Minutes

Ingredients:
- 3 tablespoons hoisin sauce
- ¼ cup honey
- 1 tablespoon soy sauce
- 3 tablespoons rice vinegar
- 2 tablespoons brown sugar
- 1½ teaspoons grated fresh ginger
- 1 to 2 teaspoons Sriracha sauce, to taste
- 2 to 3 bone-in center cut pork chops, 1-inch thick (about 1¼ pounds)
- chopped scallions, for garnish

Directions:

1. Combine the hoisin sauce, honey, soy sauce, rice vinegar, brown sugar, ginger, and Sriracha sauce in a small saucepan. Whisk the ingredients together and bring the mixture to a boil over medium-high heat on the stovetop. Reduce the heat and simmer the sauce until it has reduced in volume and thickened slightly – about 10 minutes.

2. Preheat the air fryer to 400°F.

3. Place the pork chops into the air fryer basket and pour half the hoisin BBQ sauce over the top. Air-fry for 6 minutes. Then, flip the chops over, pour the remaining hoisin BBQ sauce on top and air-fry for 6 more minutes, depending on the thickness of the pork chops. The internal temperature of the pork chops should be 155°F when tested with an instant read thermometer.

4. Let the pork chops rest for 5 minutes before serving. You can spoon a little of the sauce from the bottom drawer of the air fryer over the top if desired. Sprinkle with chopped scallions and serve.

2. Combine the pistachios, breadcrumbs, rosemary, oregano, salt and pepper in a small bowl. Drizzle in the olive oil and stir to combine.

3. Season the rack of lamb with salt and pepper on all sides and transfer it to the air fryer basket with the fat side facing up. Air-fry the lamb for 12 minutes. Remove the lamb from the air fryer and brush the fat side of the lamb rack with the Dijon mustard. Coat the rack with the pistachio mixture, pressing the breadcrumbs onto the lamb with your hands and rolling the bottom of the rack in any of the crumbs that fall off.

4. Return the rack of lamb to the air fryer and air-fry for another 3 to 7 minutes or until an instant read thermometer reads 140°F for medium. Add or subtract a couple of minutes for lamb that is more or less well cooked. (Your time will vary depending on how big the rack of lamb is.)

5. Let the lamb rest for at least 5 minutes. Then, slice into chops and serve.

Rack Of Lamb With Pistachio Crust

Servings: 2

Cooking Time: 19 Minutes

Ingredients:

- ½ cup finely chopped pistachios
- 3 tablespoons panko breadcrumbs
- 1 teaspoon chopped fresh rosemary
- 2 teaspoons chopped fresh oregano
- salt and freshly ground black pepper
- 1 tablespoon olive oil
- 1 rack of lamb, bones trimmed of fat and frenched
- 1 tablespoon Dijon mustard

Directions:

1. Preheat the air fryer to 380°F.

Pepperoni Pockets

Servings: 4
Cooking Time: 8 Minutes
Ingredients:
- 4 bread slices, 1-inch thick
- olive oil for misting
- 24 slices pepperoni (about 2 ounces)
- 1 ounce roasted red peppers, drained and patted dry
- 1 ounce Pepper Jack cheese cut into 4 slices
- pizza sauce (optional)

Directions:
1. Spray both sides of bread slices with olive oil.
2. Stand slices upright and cut a deep slit in the top to create a pocket—almost to the bottom crust but not all the way through.
3. Stuff each bread pocket with 6 slices of pepperoni, a large strip of roasted red pepper, and a slice of cheese.
4. Place bread pockets in air fryer basket, standing up. Cook at 360°F for 8 minutes, until filling is heated through and bread is lightly browned. Serve while hot as is or with pizza sauce for dipping.

Apple Cornbread Stuffed Pork Loin With Apple Gravy

Servings: 4
Cooking Time: 61 Minutes
Ingredients:
- 4 strips of bacon, chopped
- 1 Granny Smith apple, peeled, cored and finely chopped
- 2 teaspoons fresh thyme leaves
- ¼ cup chopped fresh parsley
- 2 cups cubed cornbread
- ½ cup chicken stock
- salt and freshly ground black pepper
- 1 (2-pound) boneless pork loin
- kitchen twine
- Apple Gravy:
- 2 tablespoons butter
- 1 shallot, minced
- 1 Granny Smith apple, peeled, cored and finely chopped
- 3 sprigs fresh thyme
- 2 tablespoons flour
- 1 cup chicken stock
- ½ cup apple cider
- salt and freshly ground black pepper, to taste

Directions:
1. Preheat the air fryer to 400°F.
2. Add the bacon to the air fryer and air-fry for 6 minutes until crispy. While the bacon is cooking, combine the apple, fresh thyme, parsley and cornbread in a bowl and toss well. Moisten the mixture with the chicken stock and season to taste with salt and freshly ground black pepper. Add the cooked bacon to the mixture.
3. Butterfly the pork loin by holding it flat on the cutting board with one hand, while slicing into the pork loin parallel to the cutting board with the other. Slice into the longest side of the pork loin, but stop before you cut all the way through. You should then be able to open the pork loin up like a book, making it twice as wide as it was when you started. Season the inside of the pork with salt and freshly ground black pepper.
4. Spread the cornbread mixture onto the butterflied pork loin, leaving a one-inch border around the edge of the pork. Roll the pork loin up around the stuffing to enclose the stuffing, and tie the rolled pork in several places with kitchen twine or secure with toothpicks. Try to replace

any stuffing that falls out of the roast as you roll it, by stuffing it into the ends of the rolled pork. Season the outside of the pork with salt and freshly ground black pepper.

5. Preheat the air fryer to 360°F.

6. Place the stuffed pork loin into the air fryer, seam side down. Air-fry the pork loin for 15 minutes at 360°F. Turn the pork loin over and air-fry for an additional 15 minutes. Turn the pork loin a quarter turn and air-fry for an additional 15 minutes. Turn the pork loin over again to expose the fourth side, and air-fry for an additional 10 minutes. The pork loin should register 155°F on an instant read thermometer when it is finished.

7. While the pork is cooking, make the apple gravy. Preheat a saucepan over medium heat on the stovetop and melt the butter. Add the shallot, apple and thyme sprigs and sauté until the apple starts to soften and brown a little. Add the flour and stir for a minute or two. Whisk in the stock and apple cider vigorously to prevent the flour from forming lumps. Bring the mixture to a boil to thicken and season to taste with salt and pepper.

8. Transfer the pork loin to a resting plate and loosely tent with foil, letting the pork rest for at least 5 minutes before slicing and serving with the apple gravy poured over the top.

Greek Pita Pockets

Servings: 4
Cooking Time: 7 Minutes
Ingredients:
- Dressing
- 1 cup plain yogurt
- 1 tablespoon lemon juice
- 1 teaspoon dried dill weed, crushed
- 1 teaspoon ground oregano
- ½ teaspoon salt
- Meatballs
- ½ pound ground lamb
- 1 tablespoon diced onion
- 1 teaspoon dried parsley
- 1 teaspoon dried dill weed, crushed
- ¼ teaspoon oregano
- ¼ teaspoon coriander
- ¼ teaspoon ground cumin
- ¼ teaspoon salt
- 4 pita halves
- Suggested Toppings
- red onion, slivered
- seedless cucumber, thinly sliced
- crumbled Feta cheese
- sliced black olives
- chopped fresh peppers

Directions:
1. Stir dressing ingredients together and refrigerate while preparing lamb.

2. Combine all meatball ingredients in a large bowl and stir to distribute seasonings.

3. Shape meat mixture into 12 small meatballs, rounded or slightly flattened if you prefer.

4. Cook at 390°F for 7minutes, until well done. Remove and drain on paper towels.

5. To serve, pile meatballs and your choice of toppings in pita pockets and drizzle with dressing.

Meatloaf With Tangy Tomato Glaze

Servings: 6

Cooking Time: 50 Minutes

Ingredients:

- 1 pound ground beef
- ½ pound ground pork
- ½ pound ground veal (or turkey)
- 1 medium onion, diced
- 1 small clove of garlic, minced
- 2 egg yolks, lightly beaten
- ½ cup tomato ketchup
- 1 tablespoon Worcestershire sauce
- ½ cup plain breadcrumbs*
- 2 teaspoons salt
- freshly ground black pepper
- ½ cup chopped fresh parsley, plus more for garnish
- 6 tablespoons ketchup
- 1 tablespoon balsamic vinegar
- 2 tablespoons brown sugar

Directions:

1. Combine the meats, onion, garlic, egg yolks, ketchup, Worcestershire sauce, breadcrumbs, salt, pepper and fresh parsley in a large bowl and mix well.

2. Preheat the air fryer to 350°F and pour a little water into the bottom of the air fryer drawer. (This will help prevent the grease that drips into the bottom drawer from burning and smoking.)

3. Transfer the meatloaf mixture to the air fryer basket, packing it down gently. Run a spatula around the meatloaf to create a space about ½-inch wide between the meat and the side of the air fryer basket.

4. Air-fry at 350°F for 20 minutes. Carefully invert the meatloaf onto a plate (remember to remove the basket from the air fryer drawer so you don't pour all the grease out) and slide it back into the air fryer basket to turn it over. Re-shape the meatloaf with a spatula if necessary. Air-fry for another 20 minutes at 350°F.

5. Combine the ketchup, balsamic vinegar and brown sugar in a bowl and spread the mixture over the meatloaf. Air-fry for another 10 minutes, until an instant read thermometer inserted into the center of the meatloaf registers 160°F.

6. Allow the meatloaf to rest for a few more minutes and then transfer it to a serving platter using a spatula. Slice the meatloaf, sprinkle a little chopped parsley on top if desired, and serve.

Rosemary Lamb Chops

Servings: 4

Cooking Time: 6 Minutes

Ingredients:

- 8 lamb chops
- 1 tablespoon extra-virgin olive oil
- 1 teaspoon dried rosemary, crushed
- 2 cloves garlic, minced
- 1 teaspoon sea salt
- ¼ teaspoon black pepper

Directions:

1. In a large bowl, mix together the lamb chops, olive oil, rosemary, garlic, salt, and pepper. Let sit at room temperature for 10 minutes.

2. Meanwhile, preheat the air fryer to 380°F.

3. Cook the lamb chops for 3 minutes, flip them over, and cook for another 3 minutes.

Crunchy Fried Pork Loin Chops

Servings: 3

Cooking Time: 12 Minutes

Ingredients:

- 1 cup All-purpose flour or tapioca flour
- 1 Large egg(s), well beaten
- 1½ cups Seasoned Italian-style dried bread crumbs (gluten-free, if a concern)
- 3 4- to 5-ounce boneless center-cut pork loin chops
- Vegetable oil spray

Directions:

1. Preheat the air fryer to 350°F .

2. Set up and fill three shallow soup plates or small pie plates on your counter: one for the flour, one for the beaten egg(s), and one for the bread crumbs.

3. Dredge a pork chop in the flour, coating both sides as well as around the edge. Gently shake off any excess, then dip the chop in the egg(s), again coating both sides and the edge. Let any excess egg slip back into the rest, then set the chop in the bread crumbs, turning it and pressing gently to coat well on both sides and the edge. Coat the pork chop all over with vegetable oil spray and set aside so you can dredge, coat, and spray the additional chop(s).

4. Set the chops in the basket with as much air space between them as possible. Air-fry undisturbed for 12 minutes, or until brown and crunchy and an instant-read meat thermometer inserted into the center of a chop registers 145°F.

5. Use kitchen tongs to transfer the chops to a wire rack. Cool for 5 minutes before serving.

Beef And Spinach Braciole

Servings: 4

Cooking Time: 92 Minutes

Ingredients:

- 7-inch oven-safe baking pan or casserole
- ½ onion, finely chopped
- 1 teaspoon olive oil
- ⅓ cup red wine
- 2 cups crushed tomatoes
- 1 teaspoon Italian seasoning
- ½ teaspoon garlic powder
- ¼ teaspoon crushed red pepper flakes
- 2 tablespoons chopped fresh parsley
- 2 top round steaks (about 1½ pounds)
- salt and freshly ground black pepper
- 2 cups fresh spinach, chopped
- 1 clove minced garlic
- ½ cup roasted red peppers, julienned
- ½ cup grated pecorino cheese
- ¼ cup pine nuts, toasted and rough chopped
- 2 tablespoons olive oil

Directions:

1. Preheat the air fryer to 400°F.

2. Toss the onions and olive oil together in a 7-inch metal baking pan or casserole dish. Air-fry at 400°F for 5 minutes, stirring a couple times during the cooking process. Add the red wine, crushed tomatoes, Italian seasoning, garlic powder, red pepper flakes and parsley and stir. Cover the pan tightly with aluminum foil, lower the air fryer temperature to 350°F and continue to air-fry for 15 minutes.

3. While the sauce is simmering, prepare the beef. Using a meat mallet, pound the beef until it is ¼-inch thick. Season both sides of the beef with salt and pepper. Combine the spinach, garlic, red peppers, pecorino cheese, pine nuts and olive oil in a medium bowl. Season with salt and freshly ground black pepper. Spread the mixture evenly over the steaks. Starting at one of the short

ends, roll the beef around the filling, tucking in the sides as you roll to ensure the filling is completely enclosed. Secure the beef rolls with toothpicks.

4. Remove the baking pan with the sauce from the air fryer and set it aside. Preheat the air fryer to 400°F.

5. Brush or spray the beef rolls with a little olive oil and air-fry at 400°F for 12 minutes, rotating the beef during the cooking process for even browning. When the beef is browned, submerge the rolls into the sauce in the baking pan, cover the pan with foil and return it to the air fryer. Air-fry at 250°F for 60 minutes.

6. Remove the beef rolls from the sauce. Cut each roll into slices and serve with pasta, ladling some of the sauce overtop.

Sloppy Joes

Servings: 4
Cooking Time: 17 Minutes
Ingredients:
- oil for misting or cooking spray
- 1 pound very lean ground beef
- 1 teaspoon onion powder
- ⅓ cup ketchup
- ¼ cup water
- ½ teaspoon celery seed
- 1 tablespoon lemon juice
- 1½ teaspoons brown sugar
- 1¼ teaspoons low-sodium Worcestershire sauce
- ½ teaspoon salt (optional)
- ½ teaspoon vinegar
- ⅛ teaspoon dry mustard
- hamburger or slider buns

Directions:

1. Spray air fryer basket with nonstick cooking spray or olive oil.

2. Break raw ground beef into small chunks and pile into basket.

3. Cook at 390°F for 5minutes. Stir to break apart and cook 3minutes. Stir and cook 4 minutes longer or until meat is well done.

4. Remove meat from air fryer, drain, and use a knife and fork to crumble into small pieces.

5. Give your air fryer basket a quick rinse to remove any bits of meat.

6. Place all the remaining ingredients except the buns in a 6 x 6-inch baking pan and mix together.

7. Add meat and stir well.

8. Cook at 330°F for 5minutes. Stir and cook for 2minutes.

9. Scoop onto buns.

Crispy Smoked Pork Chops

Servings: 3
Cooking Time: 8 Minutes
Ingredients:
- ⅔ cup All-purpose flour or tapioca flour
- 1 Large egg white(s)
- 2 tablespoons Water
- 1½ cups Corn flake crumbs (gluten-free, if a concern)
- 3 ½-pound, ½-inch-thick bone-in smoked pork chops

Directions:

1. Preheat the air fryer to 375°F.

2. Set up and fill three shallow soup plates or small pie plates on your counter: one for the flour; one for the egg white(s), whisked with the water until foamy; and one for the corn flake crumbs.

3. Set a chop in the flour and turn it several times, coating both sides and the edges. Gently shake off any excess flour, then set it in the beaten

egg white mixture. Turn to coat both sides as well as the edges. Let any excess egg white slip back into the rest, then set the chop in the corn flake crumbs. Turn it several times, pressing gently to coat the chop evenly on both sides and around the edge. Set the chop aside and continue coating the remaining chop(s) in the same way.

4. Set the chops in the basket with as much air space between them as possible. Air-fry undisturbed for 8 minutes, or until the coating is crunchy and the chops are heated through.

5. Use kitchen tongs to transfer the chops to a wire rack and cool for a couple of minutes before serving.

Mustard-crusted Rib-eye

Servings: 2
Cooking Time: 9 Minutes
Ingredients:
- Two 6-ounce rib-eye steaks, about 1-inch thick
- 1 teaspoon coarse salt
- ½ teaspoon coarse black pepper
- 2 tablespoons Dijon mustard

Directions:
1. Rub the steaks with the salt and pepper. Then spread the mustard on both sides of the steaks. Cover with foil and let the steaks sit at room temperature for 30 minutes.
2. Preheat the air fryer to 390°F.
3. Cook the steaks for 9 minutes. Check for an internal temperature of 140°F and immediately remove the steaks and let them rest for 5 minutes before slicing.

Lamb Chops

Servings: 2

Cooking Time: 20 Minutes
Ingredients:
- 2 teaspoons oil
- ½ teaspoon ground rosemary
- ½ teaspoon lemon juice
- 1 pound lamb chops, approximately 1-inch thick
- salt and pepper
- cooking spray

Directions:
1. Mix the oil, rosemary, and lemon juice together and rub into all sides of the lamb chops. Season to taste with salt and pepper.
2. For best flavor, cover lamb chops and allow them to rest in the fridge for 20 minutes.
3. Spray air fryer basket with nonstick spray and place lamb chops in it.
4. Cook at 360°F for approximately 20minutes. This will cook chops to medium. The meat will be juicy but have no remaining pink. Cook for a minute or two longer for well done chops. For rare chops, stop cooking after about 12minutes and check for doneness.

Lamb Meatballs With Quick Tomato Sauce

Servings: 4
Cooking Time: 8 Minutes
Ingredients:
- ½ small onion, finely diced
- 1 clove garlic, minced
- 1 pound ground lamb
- 2 tablespoons fresh parsley, finely chopped (plus more for garnish)
- 2 teaspoons fresh oregano, finely chopped
- 2 tablespoons milk
- 1 egg yolk

- salt and freshly ground black pepper
- ½ cup crumbled feta cheese, for garnish
- Tomato Sauce:
- 2 tablespoons butter
- 1 clove garlic, smashed
- pinch crushed red pepper flakes
- ¼ teaspoon ground cinnamon
- 1 (28-ounce) can crushed tomatoes
- salt, to taste

Directions:

1. Combine all ingredients for the meatballs in a large bowl and mix just until everything is combined. Shape the mixture into 1½-inch balls or shape the meat between two spoons to make quenelles (little three-sided footballs).

2. Preheat the air fryer to 400°F.

3. While the air fryer is Preheating, start the quick tomato sauce. Place the butter, garlic and red pepper flakes in a sauté pan and heat over medium heat on the stovetop. Let the garlic sizzle a little, but before the butter starts to brown, add the cinnamon and tomatoes. Bring to a simmer and simmer for 15 minutes. Season to taste with salt (but not too much as the feta that you will be sprinkling on at the end will be salty).

4. Brush the bottom of the air fryer basket with a little oil and transfer the meatballs to the air fryer basket in one layer, air-frying in batches if necessary.

5. Air-fry at 400°F for 8 minutes, giving the basket a shake once during the cooking process to turn the meatballs over.

6. To serve, spoon a pool of the tomato sauce onto plates and add the meatballs in a decorative manner. Sprinkle the feta cheese on top and garnish with more fresh parsley. Serve immediately.

Kielbasa Chunks With Pineapple & Peppers

Servings: 2
Cooking Time: 10 Minutes
Ingredients:

- ¾ pound kielbasa sausage
- 1 cup bell pepper chunks (any color)
- 1 8-ounce can pineapple chunks in juice, drained
- 1 tablespoon barbeque seasoning
- 1 tablespoon soy sauce
- cooking spray

Directions:

1. Cut sausage into ½-inch slices.

2. In a medium bowl, toss all ingredients together.

3. Spray air fryer basket with nonstick cooking spray.

4. Pour sausage mixture into the basket.

5. Cook at 390°F for approximately 5minutes. Shake basket and cook an additional 5minutes.

Honey Mesquite Pork Chops

Servings: 2
Cooking Time: 10 Minutes
Ingredients:

- 2 tablespoons mesquite seasoning
- ¼ cup honey
- 1 tablespoon olive oil
- 1 tablespoon water
- freshly ground black pepper
- 2 bone-in center cut pork chops (about 1 pound)

Directions:

1. Whisk the mesquite seasoning, honey, olive oil, water and freshly ground black pepper together in a shallow glass dish. Pierce the chops

all over and on both sides with a fork or meat tenderizer. Add the pork chops to the marinade and massage the marinade into the chops. Cover and marinate for 30 minutes.

2. Preheat the air fryer to 330°F.

3. Transfer the pork chops to the air fryer basket and pour half of the marinade over the chops, reserving the remaining marinade. Air-fry the pork chops for 6 minutes. Flip the pork chops over and pour the remaining marinade on top. Air-fry for an additional 3 minutes at 330°F. Then, increase the air fryer temperature to 400°F and air-fry the pork chops for an additional minute.

4. Transfer the pork chops to a serving plate, and let them rest for 5 minutes before serving. If you'd like a sauce for these chops, pour the cooked marinade from the bottom of the air fryer over the top.

Beef Al Carbon (street Taco Meat)

Servings: 6

Cooking Time: 8 Minutes

Ingredients:

- 1½ pounds sirloin steak, cut into ½-inch cubes
- ¾ cup lime juice
- ½ cup extra-virgin olive oil
- 1 teaspoon ground cumin
- 2 teaspoons garlic powder
- 1 teaspoon salt

Directions:

1. In a large bowl, toss together the steak, lime juice, olive oil, cumin, garlic powder, and salt. Allow the meat to marinate for 30 minutes. Drain off all the marinade and pat the meat dry with paper towels.

2. Preheat the air fryer to 400°F.

3. Place the meat in the air fryer basket and spray with cooking spray. Cook the meat for 5 minutes, toss the meat, and continue cooking another 3 minutes, until slightly crispy.

Pepper Steak

Servings: 4

Cooking Time: 30 Minutes

Ingredients:

- 2 tablespoons cornstarch
- 1 tablespoon sugar
- ¾ cup beef broth
- ¼ cup hoisin sauce
- 3 tablespoons soy sauce
- 1 teaspoon sesame oil
- ½ teaspoon freshly ground black pepper
- 1½ pounds boneless New York strip steaks, sliced into ½-inch strips
- 1 onion, sliced
- 3 small bell peppers, red, yellow and green, sliced

Directions:

1. Whisk the cornstarch and sugar together in a large bowl to break up any lumps in the cornstarch. Add the beef broth and whisk until combined and smooth. Stir in the hoisin sauce, soy sauce, sesame oil and freshly ground black pepper. Add the beef, onion and peppers, and toss to coat. Marinate the beef and vegetables at room temperature for 30 minutes, stirring a few times to keep meat and vegetables coated.

2. Preheat the air fryer to 350°F.

3. Transfer the beef, onion, and peppers to the air fryer basket with tongs, reserving the marinade. Air-fry the beef and vegetables for 30 minutes, stirring well two or three times during the cooking process.

4. While the beef is air-frying, bring the reserved marinade to a simmer in a small saucepan over medium heat on the stovetop. Simmer for 5 minutes until the sauce thickens.

5. When the steak and vegetables have finished cooking, transfer them to a serving platter. Pour the hot sauce over the pepper steak and serve with white rice.

Pork Loin

Servings: 8
Cooking Time: 50 Minutes
Ingredients:
- 1 tablespoon lime juice
- 1 tablespoon orange marmalade
- 1 teaspoon coarse brown mustard
- 1 teaspoon curry powder
- 1 teaspoon dried lemongrass
- 2-pound boneless pork loin roast
- salt and pepper
- cooking spray

Directions:
1. Mix together the lime juice, marmalade, mustard, curry powder, and lemongrass.
2. Rub mixture all over the surface of the pork loin. Season to taste with salt and pepper.
3. Spray air fryer basket with nonstick spray and place pork roast diagonally in basket.
4. Cook at 360°F for approximately 50 minutes, until roast registers 130°F on a meat thermometer.
5. Wrap roast in foil and let rest for 10minutes before slicing.

Balsamic Marinated Rib Eye Steak With Balsamic Fried Cipollini Onions

Servings: 2

Cooking Time: 22-26 Minutes
Ingredients:
- 3 tablespoons balsamic vinegar
- 2 cloves garlic, sliced
- 1 tablespoon Dijon mustard
- 1 teaspoon fresh thyme leaves
- 1 (16-ounce) boneless rib eye steak
- coarsely ground black pepper
- salt
- 1 (8-ounce) bag cipollini onions, peeled
- 1 teaspoon balsamic vinegar

Directions:
1. Combine the 3 tablespoons of balsamic vinegar, garlic, Dijon mustard and thyme in a small bowl. Pour this marinade over the steak. Pierce the steak several times with a paring knife or
2. a needle-style meat tenderizer and season it generously with coarsely ground black pepper. Flip the steak over and pierce the other side in a similar fashion, seasoning again with the coarsely ground black pepper. Marinate the steak for 2 to 24 hours in the refrigerator. When you are ready to cook, remove the steak from the refrigerator and let it sit at room temperature for 30 minutes.
3. Preheat the air fryer to 400°F.
4. Season the steak with salt and air-fry at 400°F for 12 minutes (medium-rare), 14 minutes (medium), or 16 minutes (well-done), flipping the steak once half way through the cooking time.
5. While the steak is air-frying, toss the onions with 1 teaspoon of balsamic vinegar and season with salt.
6. Remove the steak from the air fryer and let it rest while you fry the onions. Transfer the onions to the air fryer basket and air-fry for 10 minutes, adding a few more minutes if your onions are very

large. Then, slice the steak on the bias and serve with the fried onions on top.

Better-than-chinese-take-out Sesame Beef

Servings: 4

Cooking Time: 14 Minutes

Ingredients:

- 1¼ pounds Beef flank steak
- 2½ tablespoons Regular or low-sodium soy sauce or gluten-free tamari sauce
- 2 tablespoons Toasted sesame oil
- 2½ teaspoons Cornstarch
- 1 pound 2 ounces (about 4½ cups) Frozen mixed vegetables for stir-fry, thawed, seasoning packet discarded
- 3 tablespoons Unseasoned rice vinegar (see here)
- 3 tablespoons Thai sweet chili sauce
- 2 tablespoons Light brown sugar
- 2 tablespoons White sesame seeds
- 2 teaspoons Water
- Vegetable oil spray
- 1½ tablespoons Minced peeled fresh ginger
- 1 tablespoon Minced garlic

Directions:

1. Set the flank steak on a cutting board and run your clean fingers across it to figure out which way the meat's fibers are running. (Usually, they run the long way from end to end, or perhaps slightly at an angle lengthwise along the cut.) Cut the flank steak into three pieces parallel to the meat's grain. Then cut each of these pieces into ½-inch-wide strips against the grain.

2. Put the meat strips in a large bowl. For a small batch, add 2 teaspoons of the soy or tamari sauce, 2 teaspoons of the sesame oil, and ½ teaspoon of the cornstarch; for a medium batch, add 1 tablespoon of the soy or tamari sauce, 1 tablespoon of the sesame oil, and 1 teaspoon of the cornstarch; and for a large batch, add 1½ tablespoons of the soy or tamari sauce, 1½ tablespoons of the sesame oil, and 1½ teaspoons of the cornstarch. Toss well until the meat is thoroughly coated in the marinade. Set aside at room temperature.

3. Preheat the air fryer to 400°F.

4. When the machine is at temperature, place the beef strips in the basket in as close to one layer as possible. The strips will overlap or even cover each other. Air-fry for 10 minutes, tossing and rearranging the strips three times so that the covered parts get exposed, until browned and even a little crisp. Pour the strips into a clean bowl.

5. Spread the vegetables in the basket and air-fry undisturbed for 4 minutes, just until they are heated through and somewhat softened. Pour these into the bowl with the meat strips. Turn off the air fryer.

6. Whisk the rice vinegar, sweet chili sauce, brown sugar, sesame seeds, the remaining soy sauce, and the remaining sesame oil in a small bowl until well combined. For a small batch, whisk the remaining 1 teaspoon cornstarch with the water in a second small bowl to make a smooth slurry; for medium batch, whisk the remaining 1½ teaspoons cornstarch with the water in a second small bowl to make a smooth

slurry; and for a large batch, whisk the remaining 2 teaspoons cornstarch with the water in a second small bowl to make a smooth slurry.

7. Generously coat the inside of a large wok with vegetable oil spray, then set the wok over high heat for a few minutes. Add the ginger and garlic; stir-fry for 10 seconds or so, just until fragrant.

Add the meat and vegetables; stir-fry for 1 minute to heat through.

8. Add the rice vinegar mixture and continue stir-frying until the sauce is bubbling, less than 1 minute. Add the cornstarch slurry and stir-fry until the sauce has thickened, just a few seconds. Remove the wok from the heat and serve hot.

Vegetable Side Dishes Recipes

Zucchini Boats With Ham And Cheese

Servings: 4

Cooking Time: 12 Minutes

Ingredients:

- 2 6-inch-long zucchini
- 2 ounces Thinly sliced deli ham, any rind removed, meat roughly chopped
- 4 Dry-packed sun-dried tomatoes, chopped
- ⅓ cup Purchased pesto
- ¼ cup Packaged mini croutons
- ¼ cup (about 1 ounce) Shredded semi-firm mozzarella cheese

Directions:

1. Preheat the air fryer to 375°F .
2. Split the zucchini in half lengthwise and use a flatware spoon or a serrated grapefruit spoon to scoop out the insides of the halves, leaving at least a ¼-inch border all around the zucchini half. (You can save the scooped out insides to add to soups and stews—or even freeze it for a much later use.)
3. Mix the ham, sun-dried tomatoes, pesto, croutons, and half the cheese in a bowl until well combined. Pack this mixture into the zucchini "shells." Top them with the remaining cheese.
4. Set them stuffing side up in the basket without touching (even a fraction of an inch between them is enough room). Air-fry undisturbed for 12 minutes, or until softened and browned, with the cheese melted on top.
5. Use a nonstick-safe spatula to transfer the zucchini boats stuffing side up on a wire rack. Cool for 5 or 10 minutes before serving.

Yellow Squash

Servings: 4

Cooking Time: 10 Minutes

Ingredients:

- 1 large yellow squash (about 1½ cups)
- 2 eggs
- ¼ cup buttermilk
- 1 cup panko breadcrumbs
- ¼ cup white cornmeal
- ½ teaspoon salt
- oil for misting or cooking spray

Directions:

1. Preheat air fryer to 390°F.
2. Cut the squash into ¼-inch slices.
3. In a shallow dish, beat together eggs and buttermilk.
4. In sealable plastic bag or container with lid, combine ¼ cup panko crumbs, white cornmeal, and salt. Shake to mix well.
5. Place the remaining ¾ cup panko crumbs in a separate shallow dish.
6. Dump all the squash slices into the egg/buttermilk mixture. Stir to coat.
7. Remove squash from buttermilk mixture with a slotted spoon, letting excess drip off, and transfer to the panko/cornmeal mixture. Close bag or container and shake well to coat.
8. Remove squash from crumb mixture, letting excess fall off. Return squash to egg/buttermilk mixture, stirring gently to coat. If you need more liquid to coat all the squash, add a little more buttermilk.
9. Remove each squash slice from egg wash and dip in a dish of ¾ cup panko crumbs.

10. Mist squash slices with oil or cooking spray and place in air fryer basket. Squash should be in a single layer, but it's okay if the slices crowd together and overlap a little.

11. Cook at 390°F for 5minutes. Shake basket to break up any that have stuck together. Mist again with oil or spray.

12. Cook 5minutes longer and check. If necessary, mist again with oil and cook an additional two minutes, until squash slices are golden brown and crisp.

Spicy Fried Green Beans

Servings: 2

Cooking Time: 8 Minutes

Ingredients:

- 12 ounces green beans, trimmed
- 2 small dried hot red chili peppers (like árbol)
- ¼ cup panko breadcrumbs
- 1 tablespoon olive oil
- ½ teaspoon salt
- ⅛ teaspoon crushed red pepper flakes
- 2 scallions, thinly sliced

Directions:

1. Preheat the air fryer to 400°F.

2. Toss the green beans, chili peppers and panko breadcrumbs with the olive oil, salt and crushed red pepper flakes.

3. Air-fry for 8 minutes (depending on the size of the beans), shaking the basket once during the cooking process. The crumbs will fall into the bottom drawer – don't worry.

4. Transfer the green beans to a serving dish, sprinkle the scallions and the toasted crumbs from the air fryer drawer on top and serve. The dried peppers are not to be eaten, but they do look nice with the green beans. You can leave them in, or take them out as you please.

Stuffed Onions

Servings: 6

Cooking Time: 27 Minutes

Ingredients:

- 6 Small 3½- to 4-ounce yellow or white onions
- Olive oil spray
- 6 ounces Bulk sweet Italian sausage meat (gluten-free, if a concern)
- 9 Cherry tomatoes, chopped
- 3 tablespoons Seasoned Italian-style dried bread crumbs (gluten-free, if a concern)
- 3 tablespoons (about ½ ounce) Finely grated Parmesan cheese

Directions:

1. Preheat the air fryer to 325°F (or 330°F, if that's the closest setting).

2. Cut just enough off the root ends of the onions so they will stand up on a cutting board when this end is turned down. Carefully peel off just the brown, papery skin. Now cut the top quarter off each and place the onion back on the cutting board with this end facing up. Use a flatware spoon (preferably a serrated grapefruit spoon) or a melon baller to scoop out the "insides" (interior layers) of the onion, leaving enough of the bottom and side walls so that the onion does not collapse. Depending on the thickness of the layers in the onion, this may be one or two of those layers—or even three, if they're very thin.

3. Coat the insides and outsides of the onions with olive oil spray. Set the onion "shells" in the basket and air-fry for 15 minutes.

4. Meanwhile, make the filling. Set a medium skillet over medium heat for a couple of minutes, then crumble in the sausage meat. Cook, stirring often, until browned, about 4 minutes. Transfer

the contents of the skillet to a medium bowl (leave the fat behind in the skillet or add it to the bowl, depending on your cross-trainer regimen). Stir in the tomatoes, bread crumbs, and cheese until well combined.

5. When the onions are ready, use a nonstick-safe spatula to gently transfer them to a cutting board. Increase the air fryer's temperature to 350°F .

6. Pack the sausage mixture into the onion shells, gently compacting the filling and mounding it up at the top.

7. When the machine is at temperature, set the onions stuffing side up in the basket with at least ¼ inch between them. Air-fry for 12 minutes, or until lightly browned and sizzling hot.

8. Use a nonstick-safe spatula, and perhaps a flatware fork for balance, to transfer the onions to a cutting board or serving platter. Cool for 5 minutes before serving.

Moroccan Cauliflower

Servings: 6
Cooking Time: 15 Minutes
Ingredients:
- 1 tablespoon curry powder
- 2 teaspoons smoky paprika
- ½ teaspoon ground cumin
- ½ teaspoon salt
- 1 head cauliflower, cut into bite-size pieces
- ¼ cup red wine vinegar
- 2 tablespoons extra-virgin olive oil
- 2 tablespoons chopped parsley

Directions:
1. Preheat the air fryer to 370°F.
2. In a large bowl, mix the curry powder, paprika, cumin, and salt. Add the cauliflower and stir to coat. Pour the red wine vinegar over the top and continue stirring.

3. Place the cauliflower into the air fryer basket; drizzle olive oil over the top.

4. Cook the cauliflower for 5 minutes, toss, and cook another 5 minutes. Raise the temperature to 400°F and continue cooking for 4 to 6 minutes, or until crispy.

Chicken Eggrolls

Servings: 10
Cooking Time: 17 Minutes
Ingredients:
- 1 tablespoon vegetable oil
- ¼ cup chopped onion
- 1 clove garlic, minced
- 1 cup shredded carrot
- ½ cup thinly sliced celery
- 2 cups cooked chicken
- 2 cups shredded white cabbage
- ½ cup teriyaki sauce
- 20 egg roll wrappers
- 1 egg, whisked
- 1 tablespoon water

Directions:
1. Preheat the air fryer to 390°F.
2. In a large skillet, heat the oil over medium-high heat. Add in the onion and sauté for 1 minute. Add in the garlic and sauté for 30 seconds. Add in the carrot and celery and cook for 2 minutes. Add in the chicken, cabbage, and teriyaki sauce. Allow the mixture to cook for 1 minute, stirring to combine. Remove from the heat.

3. In a small bowl, whisk together the egg and water for brushing the edges.

4. Lay the eggroll wrappers out at an angle. Place ¼ cup filling in the center. Fold the bottom

corner up first and then fold in the corners; roll up to complete eggroll.

5. Place the eggrolls in the air fryer basket, spray with cooking spray, and cook for 8 minutes, turn over, and cook another 2 to 4 minutes.

Mushrooms

Servings: 4
Cooking Time: 12 Minutes

Ingredients:
- 8 ounces whole white button mushrooms
- ½ teaspoon salt
- ⅛ teaspoon pepper
- ¼ teaspoon garlic powder
- ¼ teaspoon onion powder
- 5 tablespoons potato starch
- 1 egg, beaten
- ¾ cup panko breadcrumbs
- oil for misting or cooking spray

Directions:
1. Place mushrooms in a large bowl. Add the salt, pepper, garlic and onion powders, and stir well to distribute seasonings.

2. Add potato starch to mushrooms and toss in bowl until well coated.

3. Dip mushrooms in beaten egg, roll in panko crumbs, and mist with oil or cooking spray.

4. Place mushrooms in air fryer basket. You can cook them all at once, and it's okay if a few are stacked.

5. Cook at 390°F for 5minutes. Shake basket, then continue cooking for 7 more minutes, until golden brown and crispy.

Home Fries

Servings: 4
Cooking Time: 20 Minutes

Ingredients:
- 3 pounds potatoes, cut into 1-inch cubes
- ½ teaspoon oil
- salt and pepper

Directions:
1. In a large bowl, mix the potatoes and oil thoroughly.

2. Cook at 390°F for 10minutes and shake the basket to redistribute potatoes.

3. Cook for an additional 10 minutes, until brown and crisp.

4. Season with salt and pepper to taste.

Onion Rings

Servings: 4
Cooking Time: 12 Minutes

Ingredients:
- 1 large onion (preferably Vidalia or 1015)
- ½ cup flour, plus 2 tablespoons
- ½ teaspoon salt
- ½ cup beer, plus 2 tablespoons
- 1 cup crushed panko breadcrumbs
- oil for misting or cooking spray

Directions:
1. Peel onion, slice, and separate into rings.

2. In a large bowl, mix together the flour and salt. Add beer and stir until it stops foaming and makes a thick batter.

3. Place onion rings in batter and stir to coat.

4. Place breadcrumbs in a sealable plastic bag or container with lid.

5. Working with a few at a time, remove onion rings from batter, shaking off excess, and drop into breadcrumbs. Shake to coat, then lay out onion rings on cookie sheet or wax paper.

6. When finished, spray onion rings with oil or cooking spray and pile into air fryer basket.

7. Cook at 390°F for 5minutes. Shake basket and mist with oil. Cook 5minutes and mist again. Cook an additional 2 minutes, until golden brown and crispy.

Shoestring Butternut Squash Fries

Servings: 3
Cooking Time: 16 Minutes
Ingredients:
- 1 pound 2 ounces Spiralized butternut squash strands
- Vegetable oil spray
- To taste Coarse sea salt or kosher salt

Directions:
1. Preheat the air fryer to 375°F .
2. Place the spiralized squash in a big bowl. Coat the strands with vegetable oil spray, toss well, coat again, and toss several times to make sure all the strands have been oiled.
3. When the machine is at temperature, pour the strands into the basket and spread them out into as even a layer as possible. Air-fry for 16 minutes, tossing and rearranging the strands every 4 minutes, or until they're lightly browned and crisp.
4. Pour the contents of the basket into a serving bowl, add salt to taste, and toss well before serving hot.

Sweet Potato Fries

Servings: 4
Cooking Time: 30 Minutes
Ingredients:
- 2 pounds sweet potatoes
- 1 teaspoon dried marjoram
- 2 teaspoons olive oil
- sea salt

Directions:
1. Peel and cut the potatoes into ¼-inch sticks, 4 to 5 inches long.
2. In a sealable plastic bag or bowl with lid, toss sweet potatoes with marjoram and olive oil. Rub seasonings in to coat well.
3. Pour sweet potatoes into air fryer basket and cook at 390°F for approximately 30 minutes, until cooked through with some brown spots on edges.
4. Season to taste with sea salt.

Roasted Garlic And Thyme Tomatoes

Servings: 2
Cooking Time: 15 Minutes
Ingredients:
- 4 Roma tomatoes
- 1 tablespoon olive oil
- salt and freshly ground black pepper
- 1 clove garlic, minced
- ½ teaspoon dried thyme

Directions:
1. Preheat the air fryer to 390°F.
2. Cut the tomatoes in half and scoop out the seeds and any pithy parts with your fingers. Place the tomatoes in a bowl and toss with the olive oil, salt, pepper, garlic and thyme.
3. Transfer the tomatoes to the air fryer, cut side up. Air-fry for 15 minutes. The edges should just start to brown. Let the tomatoes cool to an edible temperature for a few minutes and then use in pastas, on top of crostini, or as an accompaniment to any poultry, meat or fish.

Roasted Heirloom Carrots With Orange And Thyme

Servings: 2

Cooking Time: 12 Minutes

Ingredients:

- 10 to 12 heirloom or rainbow carrots (about 1 pound), scrubbed but not peeled
- 1 teaspoon olive oil
- salt and freshly ground black pepper
- 1 tablespoon butter
- 1 teaspoon fresh orange zest
- 1 teaspoon chopped fresh thyme

Directions:

1. Preheat the air fryer to 400°F.

2. Scrub the carrots and halve them lengthwise. Toss them in the olive oil, season with salt and freshly ground black pepper and transfer to the air fryer.

3. Air-fry at 400°F for 12 minutes, shaking the basket every once in a while to rotate the carrots as they cook.

4. As soon as the carrots have finished cooking, add the butter, orange zest and thyme and toss all the ingredients together in the air fryer basket to melt the butter and coat evenly. Serve warm.

Sweet Potato Curly Fries

Servings: 4

Cooking Time: 10 Minutes

Ingredients:

- 2 medium sweet potatoes, washed
- 2 tablespoons avocado oil
- ¾ teaspoon salt, divided
- 1 medium avocado
- ½ teaspoon garlic powder
- ½ teaspoon paprika
- ¼ teaspoon black pepper
- ½ juice lime
- 3 tablespoons fresh cilantro

Directions:

1. Preheat the air fryer to 400°F.

2. Using a spiralizer, create curly spirals with the sweet potatoes. Keep the pieces about 1½ inches long. Continue until all the potatoes are used.

3. In a large bowl, toss the curly sweet potatoes with the avocado oil and ½ teaspoon of the salt.

4. Place the potatoes in the air fryer basket and cook for 5 minutes; shake and cook another 5 minutes.

5. While cooking, add the avocado, garlic, paprika, pepper, the remaining ¼ teaspoon of salt, lime juice, and cilantro to a blender and process until smooth. Set aside.

6. When cooking completes, remove the fries and serve warm with the lime avocado sauce.

Roman Artichokes

Servings: 4

Cooking Time: 12 Minutes

Ingredients:

- 2 9-ounce box(es) frozen artichoke heart quarters, thawed
- 1½ tablespoons Olive oil
- 2 teaspoons Minced garlic
- 1 teaspoon Table salt
- Up to ½ teaspoon Red pepper flakes

Directions:

1. Preheat the air fryer to 400°F.

2. Gently toss the artichoke heart quarters, oil, garlic, salt, and red pepper flakes in a bowl until the quarters are well coated.

3. When the machine is at temperature, scrape the contents of the bowl into the basket. Spread the artichoke heart quarters out into as close to one layer as possible. Air-fry undisturbed for 8

minutes. Gently toss and rearrange the quarters so that any covered or touching parts are now exposed to the air currents, then air-fry undisturbed for 4 minutes more, until very crisp.

4. Gently pour the contents of the basket onto a wire rack. Cool for a few minutes before serving.

Jerk Rubbed Corn On The Cob

Servings: 4
Cooking Time: 6 Minutes

Ingredients:
- 1 teaspoon ground allspice
- 1 teaspoon dried thyme
- ½ teaspoon ground ginger
- ½ teaspoon ground cinnamon
- ¼ teaspoon ground nutmeg
- ⅛ teaspoon ground cayenne pepper
- 1 teaspoon salt
- 2 tablespoons butter, melted
- 4 ears of corn, husked

Directions:
1. Preheat the air fryer to 380°F.
2. Combine all the spices in a bowl. Brush the corn with the melted butter and then sprinkle the spices generously on all sides of each ear of corn.
3. Transfer the ears of corn to the air fryer basket. It's ok if they are crisscrossed on top of each other. Air-fry at 380°F for 6 minutes, rotating the ears as they cook.
4. Brush more butter on at the end and sprinkle with any remaining spice mixture.

Butternut Medallions With Honey Butter And Sage

Servings: 2
Cooking Time: 15 Minutes

Ingredients:
- 1 butternut squash, peeled
- olive oil, in a spray bottle
- salt and freshly ground black pepper
- 2 tablespoons butter, softened
- 2 tablespoons honey
- pinch ground cinnamon
- pinch ground nutmeg
- chopped fresh sage

Directions:
1. Preheat the air fryer to 370°F.
2. Cut the neck of the butternut squash into disks about ½-inch thick. (Use the base of the butternut squash for another use.) Brush or spray the disks with oil and season with salt and freshly ground black pepper.
3. Transfer the butternut disks to the air fryer in one layer (or just ever so slightly overlapping). Air-fry at 370°F for 5 minutes.
4. While the butternut squash is cooking, combine the butter, honey, cinnamon and nutmeg in a small bowl. Brush this mixture on the butternut squash, flip the disks over and brush the other side as well. Continue to air-fry at 370°F for another 5 minutes. Flip the disks once more, brush with more of the honey butter and air-fry for another 5 minutes. The butternut should be browning nicely around the edges.
5. Remove the butternut squash from the air-fryer and repeat with additional batches if necessary. Transfer to a serving platter, sprinkle with the fresh sage and serve.

Roasted Broccoli And Red Bean Salad

Servings: 3

Cooking Time: 14 Minutes

Ingredients:

- 3 cups (about 1 pound) 1- to 1½-inch fresh broccoli florets (not frozen)
- 1½ tablespoons Olive oil spray
- 1¼ cups Canned red kidney beans, drained and rinsed
- 3 tablespoons Minced yellow or white onion
- 2 tablespoons plus 1 teaspoon Red wine vinegar
- ¾ teaspoon Dried oregano
- ¼ teaspoon Table salt
- ¼ teaspoon Ground black pepper

Directions:

1. Preheat the air fryer to 375°F .

2. Put the broccoli florets in a big bowl, coat them generously with olive oil spray, then toss to coat all surfaces, even down into the crannies, spraying them a couple of times more.

3. Pour the florets into the basket, spreading them into as close to one layer as you can. Air-fry for 12 minutes, tossing and rearranging the florets twice so that any touching or covered parts are eventually exposed to the air currents, until light browned but still a bit firm. (If the machine is at 360°F, you may need to add 2 minutes to the cooking time.)

4. Dump the contents of the basket onto a large cutting board. Cool for a minute or two, then chop the florets into small bits. Scrape these into a bowl and add the kidney beans, onion, vinegar, oregano, salt, and pepper. Toss well and serve warm or at room temperature.

Salmon Salad With Steamboat Dressing

Servings: 4

Cooking Time: 18 Minutes

Ingredients:

- ¼ teaspoon salt
- 1½ teaspoons dried dill weed
- 1 tablespoon fresh lemon juice
- 8 ounces fresh or frozen salmon fillet (skin on)
- 8 cups shredded romaine, Boston, or other leaf lettuce
- 8 spears cooked asparagus, cut in 1-inch pieces
- 8 cherry tomatoes, halved or quartered

Directions:

1. Mix the salt and dill weed together. Rub the lemon juice over the salmon on both sides and sprinkle the dill and salt all over. Refrigerate for 15 to 20minutes.

2. Make Steamboat Dressing and refrigerate while cooking salmon and preparing salad.

3. Cook salmon in air fryer basket at 330°F for 18 minutes. Cooking time will vary depending on thickness of fillets. When done, salmon should flake with fork but still be moist and tender.

4. Remove salmon from air fryer and cool slightly. At this point, the skin should slide off easily. Cut salmon into 4 pieces and discard skin.

5. Divide the lettuce among 4 plates. Scatter asparagus spears and tomato pieces evenly over the lettuce, allowing roughly 2 whole spears and 2 whole cherry tomatoes per plate.

6. Top each salad with one portion of the salmon and drizzle with a tablespoon of dressing. Serve with additional dressing to pass at the table.

Roasted Ratatouille Vegetables

Servings: 2

Cooking Time: 15 Minutes

Ingredients:

- 1 baby or Japanese eggplant, cut into 1½-inch cubes
- 1 red pepper, cut into 1-inch chunks
- 1 yellow pepper, cut into 1-inch chunks
- 1 zucchini, cut into 1-inch chunks
- 1 clove garlic, minced
- ½ teaspoon dried basil
- 1 tablespoon olive oil
- salt and freshly ground black pepper
- ¼ cup sliced sun-dried tomatoes in oil
- 2 tablespoons chopped fresh basil

Directions:

1. Preheat the air fryer to 400°F.

2. Toss the eggplant, peppers and zucchini with the garlic, dried basil, olive oil, salt and freshly ground black pepper.

3. Air-fry the vegetables at 400°F for 15 minutes, shaking the basket a few times during the cooking process to redistribute the ingredients.

4. As soon as the vegetables are tender, toss them with the sliced sun-dried tomatoes and fresh basil and serve.

Crispy, Cheesy Leeks

Servings: 4

Cooking Time: 15 Minutes

Ingredients:

- 2 Medium leek(s), about 9 ounces each
- Olive oil spray
- ¼ cup Seasoned Italian-style dried bread crumbs (gluten-free, if a concern)
- ¼ cup (about ¾ ounce) Finely grated Parmesan cheese
- 2 tablespoons Olive oil

Directions:

1. Preheat the air fryer to 350°F .

2. Trim off the root end of the leek(s) as well as the dark green top(s), leaving about a 5-inch usable section. Split the leek section(s) in half lengthwise. Set the leek halves cut side up on your work surface. Pull out and remove in one piece the semicircles that make up the inner structure of the leek, about halfway down. Set the removed "inside" next to the outer leek "shells" on your cutting board. Generously coat them all on all sides (particularly the "bottoms") with olive oil spray.

3. Set the leeks and their insides cut side up in the basket with as much air space between them as possible. Air-fry undisturbed for 12 minutes.

4. Meanwhile, mix the bread crumbs, cheese, and olive oil in a small bowl until well combined.

5. After 12 minutes in the air fryer, sprinkle this mixture inside the leek shells and on top of the leek insides. Increase the machine's temperature to 375°F (or 380°F or 390°F, if one of these is the closest setting). Air-fry undisturbed for 3 minutes, or until the topping is lightly browned.

6. Use a nonstick-safe spatula to transfer the leeks to a serving platter. Cool for a few minutes before serving warm.

Fried Pearl Onions With Balsamic Vinegar And Basil

Servings: 2

Cooking Time: 10 Minutes

Ingredients:

- 1 pound fresh pearl onions
- 1 tablespoon olive oil
- salt and freshly ground black pepper
- 1 teaspoon high quality aged balsamic vinegar
- 1 tablespoon chopped fresh basil leaves (or mint)

Directions:

1. Preheat the air fryer to 400°F.

2. Decide whether you want to peel the onions before or after they cook. Peeling them ahead of time is a little more laborious. Peeling after they cook is easier, but a little messier since the onions are hot and you may discard more of the onion than you'd like to. If you opt to peel them first, trim the tiny root of the onions off and pinch off any loose papery skins. (It's ok if there are some skins left on the onions.) Toss the pearl onions with the olive oil, salt and freshly ground black pepper.

3. Air-fry for 10 minutes, shaking the basket a couple of times during the cooking process. (If your pearl onions are very large, you may need to add a couple of minutes to this cooking time.)

4. Let the onions cool slightly and then slip off any remaining skins.

5. Toss the onions with the balsamic vinegar and basil and serve.

Bacon-wrapped Asparagus

Servings: 4

Cooking Time: 10 Minutes

Ingredients:

- 1 tablespoon extra-virgin olive oil
- ½ teaspoon sea salt
- ¼ cup grated Parmesan cheese
- 1 pound asparagus, ends trimmed
- 8 slices bacon

Directions:

1. Preheat the air fryer to 380°F.

2. In large bowl, mix together the olive oil, sea salt, and Parmesan cheese. Toss the asparagus in the olive oil mixture.

3. Evenly divide the asparagus into 8 bundles. Wrap 1 piece of bacon around each bundle, not overlapping the bacon but spreading it across the bundle.

4. Place the asparagus bundles into the air fryer basket, not touching. Work in batches as needed.

5. Cook for 8 minutes; check for doneness, and cook another 2 minutes.

Asparagus

Servings: 4

Cooking Time: 9 Minutes

Ingredients:

- 1 bunch asparagus (approx. 1 pound), washed and trimmed
- ⅛ teaspoon dried tarragon, crushed
- salt and pepper
- 1 to 2 teaspoons extra-light olive oil

Directions:

1. Spread asparagus spears on cookie sheet or cutting board.

2. Sprinkle with tarragon, salt, and pepper.

3. Drizzle with 1 teaspoon of oil and roll the spears or mix by hand. If needed, add up to 1 more teaspoon of oil and mix again until all spears are lightly coated.

4. Place spears in air fryer basket. If necessary, bend the longer spears to make them fit. It doesn't matter if they don't lie flat.

5. Cook at 390°F for 5minutes. Shake basket or stir spears with a spoon.

6. Cook for an additional 4 minutes or just until crisp-tender.

Cheesy Potato Skins

Servings: 6

Cooking Time: 54 Minutes

Ingredients:

- 3 6- to 8-ounce small russet potatoes
- 3 Thick-cut bacon strips, halved widthwise (gluten-free, if a concern)
- ¾ teaspoon Mild paprika
- ¼ teaspoon Garlic powder
- ¼ teaspoon Table salt
- ¼ teaspoon Ground black pepper
- ½ cup plus 1 tablespoon (a little over 2 ounces) Shredded Cheddar cheese
- 3 tablespoons Thinly sliced trimmed chives
- 6 tablespoons (a little over 1 ounce) Finely grated Parmesan cheese

Directions:

1. Preheat the air fryer to 375°F .

2. Prick each potato in four places with a fork (not four places in a line but four places all around the potato). Set the potatoes in the basket with as much air space between them as possible. Air-fry undisturbed for 45 minutes, or until the potatoes are tender when pricked with a fork.

3. Use kitchen tongs to gently transfer the potatoes to a wire rack. Cool for 15 minutes. Maintain the machine's temperature.

4. Lay the bacon strip halves in the basket in one layer. They may touch but should not overlap. Air-fry undisturbed for 5 minutes, until crisp. Use those same tongs to transfer the bacon pieces to the wire rack. If there's a great deal of rendered bacon fat in the basket's bottom or on a tray under the basket attachment, pour this into a bowl, cool, and discard. Don't throw it down the drain!

5. Cut the potatoes in half lengthwise (not just slit them open but actually cut in half). Use a flatware spoon to scoop the hot, soft middles into a bowl, leaving ½ inch of potato all around the inside of the spud next to the skin. Sprinkle the inside of the potato "shells" evenly with paprika, garlic powder, salt, and pepper.

6. Chop the bacon pieces into small bits. Sprinkle these along with the Cheddar and chives evenly inside the potato shells. Crumble 2 to 3 tablespoons of the soft potato insides over the filling mixture. Divide the grated Parmesan evenly over the tops of the potatoes.

7. Set the stuffed potatoes in the basket with as much air space between them as possible. Air-fry undisturbed for 4 minutes, until the cheese melts and lightly browns.

8. Use kitchen tongs to gently transfer the stuffed potato halves to a wire rack. Cool for 5 minutes before serving.

Glazed Carrots

Servings: 4

Cooking Time: 10 Minutes

Ingredients:

- 2 teaspoons honey
- 1 teaspoon orange juice
- ½ teaspoon grated orange rind
- ⅛ teaspoon ginger
- 1 pound baby carrots
- 2 teaspoons olive oil
- ¼ teaspoon salt

Directions:

1. Combine honey, orange juice, grated rind, and ginger in a small bowl and set aside.

2. Toss the carrots, oil, and salt together to coat well and pour them into the air fryer basket.

3. Cook at 390°F for 5minutes. Shake basket to stir a little and cook for 4 minutes more, until carrots are barely tender.

4. Pour carrots into air fryer baking pan.

5. Stir the honey mixture to combine well, pour glaze over carrots, and stir to coat.

6. Cook at 360°F for 1 minute or just until heated through.

Blistered Green Beans

Servings: 3

Cooking Time: 10 Minutes

Ingredients:

- ¾ pound Green beans, trimmed on both ends
- 1½ tablespoons Olive oil
- 3 tablespoons Pine nuts
- 1½ tablespoons Balsamic vinegar
- 1½ teaspoons Minced garlic
- ¾ teaspoon Table salt
- ¾ teaspoon Ground black pepper

Directions:

1. Preheat the air fryer to 400°F.

2. Toss the green beans and oil in a large bowl until all the green beans are glistening.

3. When the machine is at temperature, pile the green beans into the basket. Air-fry for 10 minutes, tossing often to rearrange the green beans in the basket, or until blistered and tender.

4. Dump the contents of the basket into a serving bowl. Add the pine nuts, vinegar, garlic, salt, and pepper. Toss well to coat and combine. Serve warm or at room temperature.

Buttery Rolls

Servings: 6

Cooking Time: 14 Minutes

Ingredients:

- 6½ tablespoons Room-temperature whole or low-fat milk
- 3 tablespoons plus 1 teaspoon Butter, melted and cooled
- 3 tablespoons plus 1 teaspoon (or 1 medium egg, well beaten) Pasteurized egg substitute, such as Egg Beaters
- 1½ tablespoons Granulated white sugar
- 1¼ teaspoons Instant yeast
- ¼ teaspoon Table salt
- 2 cups, plus more for dusting All-purpose flour
- Vegetable oil
- Additional melted butter, for brushing

Directions:

1. Stir the milk, melted butter, pasteurized egg substitute (or whole egg), sugar, yeast, and salt in a medium bowl to combine. Stir in the flour just until the mixture makes a soft dough.

2. Lightly flour a clean, dry work surface. Turn the dough out onto the work surface. Knead the dough for 5 minutes to develop the gluten.

3. Lightly oil the inside of a clean medium bowl. Gather the dough into a compact ball and set it in the bowl. Turn the dough over so that its surface has oil on it all over. Cover the bowl tightly with plastic wrap and set aside in a warm, draft-free place until the dough has doubled in bulk, about 1½ hours.

4. Punch down the dough, then turn it out onto a clean, dry work surface. Divide it into 5 even balls for a small batch, 6 balls for a medium batch, or 8 balls for a large one.

5. For a small batch, lightly oil the inside of a 6-inch round cake pan and set the balls around its perimeter, separating them as much as possible.

6. For a medium batch, lightly oil the inside of a 7-inch round cake pan and set the balls in it with one ball at its center, separating them as much as possible.

7. For a large batch, lightly oil the inside of an 8-inch round cake pan and set the balls in it with one at the center, separating them as much as possible.

8. Cover with plastic wrap and set aside to rise for 30 minutes.

9. Preheat the air fryer to 350°F .

10. Uncover the pan and brush the rolls with a little melted butter, perhaps ½ teaspoon per roll. When the machine is at temperature, set the cake pan in the basket. Air-fry undisturbed for 14 minutes, or until the rolls have risen and browned.

11. Using kitchen tongs and a nonstick-safe spatula, two hot pads, or silicone baking mitts, transfer the cake pan from the basket to a wire rack. Cool the rolls in the pan for a minute or two. Turn the rolls out onto a wire rack, set them top side up again, and cool for at least another couple of minutes before serving warm.

Asiago Broccoli

Servings: 4

Cooking Time: 14 Minutes

Ingredients:

- 1 head broccoli, cut into florets
- 1 tablespoon extra-virgin olive oil
- 1 teaspoon minced garlic
- ¼ teaspoon ground black pepper
- ¼ teaspoon salt
- ¼ cup asiago cheese

Directions:

1. Preheat the air fryer to 360°F.

2. In a medium bowl, toss the broccoli florets with the olive oil, garlic, pepper, and salt. Lightly spray the air fryer basket with olive oil spray.

3. Place the broccoli florets into the basket and cook for 7 minutes. Shake the basket and sprinkle the broccoli with cheese. Cook another 7 minutes.

4. Remove from the basket and serve warm.

Curried Cauliflower With Cashews And Yogurt

Servings: 2

Cooking Time: 12 Minutes

Ingredients:

- 4 cups cauliflower florets (about half a large head)
- 1 tablespoon olive oil
- salt
- 1 teaspoon curry powder
- ½ cup toasted, chopped cashews
- Cool Yogurt Drizzle
- ¼ cup plain yogurt
- 2 tablespoons sour cream
- 1 teaspoon lemon juice
- pinch cayenne pepper
- salt
- 1 teaspoon honey
- 1 tablespoon chopped fresh cilantro, plus leaves for garnish

Directions:

1. Preheat the air fryer to 400°F.

2. Toss the cauliflower florets with the olive oil, salt and curry powder, coating evenly.

3. Transfer the cauliflower to the air fryer basket and air-fry at 400°F for 12 minutes, shaking the basket a couple of times during the cooking process.

4. While the cauliflower is cooking, make the cool yogurt drizzle by combining all ingredients in a bowl.

5. When the cauliflower is cooked to your liking, serve it warm with the cool yogurt either underneath or drizzled over the top. Scatter the cashews and cilantro leaves around.

Desserts And Sweets

Peach Cobbler

Servings: 4
Cooking Time: 12 Minutes
Ingredients:

- 16 ounces frozen peaches, thawed, with juice (do not drain)
- 6 tablespoons sugar
- 1 tablespoon cornstarch
- 1 tablespoon water
- Crust
- ½ cup flour
- ¼ teaspoon salt
- 3 tablespoons butter
- 1½ tablespoons cold water
- ¼ teaspoon sugar

Directions:

1. Place peaches, including juice, and sugar in air fryer baking pan. Stir to mix well.
2. In a small cup, dissolve cornstarch in the water. Stir into peaches.
3. In a medium bowl, combine the flour and salt. Cut in butter using knives or a pastry blender. Stir in the cold water to make a stiff dough.
4. On a floured board or wax paper, pat dough into a square or circle slightly smaller than your air fryer baking pan. Cut diagonally into 4 pieces.
5. Place dough pieces on top of peaches, leaving a tiny bit of space between the edges. Sprinkle very lightly with sugar, no more than about ¼ teaspoon.
6. Cook at 360°F for 12 minutes, until fruit bubbles and crust browns.

Glazed Cherry Turnovers

Servings: 8
Cooking Time: 14 Minutes
Ingredients:

- 2 sheets frozen puff pastry, thawed
- 1 (21-ounce) can premium cherry pie filling
- 2 teaspoons ground cinnamon
- 1 egg, beaten
- 1 cup sliced almonds
- 1 cup powdered sugar
- 2 tablespoons milk

Directions:

1. Roll a sheet of puff pastry out into a square that is approximately 10-inches by 10-inches. Cut this large square into quarters.
2. Mix the cherry pie filling and cinnamon together in a bowl. Spoon ¼ cup of the cherry filling into the center of each puff pastry square. Brush the perimeter of the pastry square with the egg wash. Fold one corner of the puff pastry over the cherry pie filling towards the opposite corner, forming a triangle. Seal the two edges of the pastry together with the tip of a fork, making a design with the tines. Brush the top of the turnovers with the egg wash and sprinkle sliced almonds over each one. Repeat these steps with the second sheet of puff pastry. You should have eight turnovers at the end.
3. Preheat the air fryer to 370°F.
4. Air-fry two turnovers at a time for 14 minutes, carefully turning them over halfway through the cooking time.
5. While the turnovers are cooking, make the glaze by whisking the powdered sugar and milk together in a small bowl until smooth. Let the glaze sit for a minute so the sugar can absorb the milk. If the consistency is still too thick to drizzle,

add a little more milk, a drop at a time, and stir until smooth.

6. Let the cooked cherry turnovers sit for at least 10 minutes. Then drizzle the glaze over each turnover in a zigzag motion. Serve warm or at room temperature.

Mixed Berry Hand Pies

Servings: 4
Cooking Time: 15 Minutes
Ingredients:
- ¾ cup sugar
- ½ teaspoon ground cinnamon
- 1 tablespoon cornstarch
- 1 cup blueberries
- 1 cup blackberries
- 1 cup raspberries, divided
- 1 teaspoon water
- 1 package refrigerated pie dough (or your own homemade pie dough)
- 1 egg, beaten

Directions:
1. Combine the sugar, cinnamon, and cornstarch in a small saucepan. Add the blueberries, blackberries, and ½ cup of the raspberries. Toss the berries gently to coat them evenly. Add the teaspoon of water to the saucepan and turn the stovetop on to medium-high heat, stirring occasionally. Once the berries break down, release their juice and start to simmer (about 5 minutes), simmer for another couple of minutes and then transfer the mixture to a bowl, stir in the remaining ½ cup of raspberries and let it cool.
2. Preheat the air fryer to 370°F.
3. Cut the pie dough into four 5-inch circles and four 6-inch circles.

4. Spread the 6-inch circles on a flat surface. Divide the berry filling between all four circles. Brush the perimeter of the dough circles with a little water. Place the 5-inch circles on top of the filling and press the perimeter of the dough circles together to seal. Roll the edges of the bottom circle up over the top circle to make a crust around the filling. Press a fork around the crust to make decorative indentations and to seal the crust shut. Brush the pies with egg wash and sprinkle a little sugar on top. Poke a small hole in the center of each pie with a paring knife to vent the dough.
5. Air-fry two pies at a time. Brush or spray the air fryer basket with oil and place the pies into the basket. Air-fry for 9 minutes. Turn the pies over and air-fry for another 6 minutes. Serve warm or at room temperature.

Molten Chocolate Almond Cakes

Servings: 3
Cooking Time: 13 Minutes
Ingredients:
- butter and flour for the ramekins
- 4 ounces bittersweet chocolate, chopped
- ½ cup (1 stick) unsalted butter
- 2 eggs
- 2 egg yolks
- ¼ cup sugar
- ½ teaspoon pure vanilla extract, or almond extract
- 1 tablespoon all-purpose flour
- 3 tablespoons ground almonds
- 8 to 12 semisweet chocolate discs (or 4 chunks of chocolate)
- cocoa powder or powdered sugar, for dusting
- toasted almonds, coarsely chopped

Directions:

1. Butter and flour three (6-ounce) ramekins. (Butter the ramekins and then coat the butter with flour by shaking it around in the ramekin and dumping out any excess.)

2. Melt the chocolate and butter together, either in the microwave or in a double boiler. In a separate bowl, beat the eggs, egg yolks and sugar together until light and smooth. Add the vanilla extract. Whisk the chocolate mixture into the egg mixture. Stir in the flour and ground almonds.

3. Preheat the air fryer to 330°F.

4. Transfer the batter carefully to the buttered ramekins, filling halfway. Place two or three chocolate discs in the center of the batter and then fill the ramekins to ½-inch below the top with the remaining batter. Place the ramekins into the air fryer basket and air-fry at 330°F for 13 minutes. The sides of the cake should be set, but the centers should be slightly soft. Remove the ramekins from the air fryer and let the cakes sit for 5 minutes. (If you'd like the cake a little less molten, air-fry for 14 minutes and let the cakes sit for 4 minutes.)

5. Run a butter knife around the edge of the ramekins and invert the cakes onto a plate. Lift the ramekin off the plate slowly and carefully so that the cake doesn't break. Dust with cocoa powder or powdered sugar and serve with a scoop of ice cream and some coarsely chopped toasted almonds.

Giant Vegan Chocolate Chip Cookie

Servings: 4
Cooking Time: 16 Minutes
Ingredients:
- ⅔ cup All-purpose flour
- 5 tablespoons Rolled oats (not quick-cooking or steel-cut oats)
- ¼ teaspoon Baking soda
- ¼ teaspoon Table salt
- 5 tablespoons Granulated white sugar
- ¼ cup Vegetable oil
- 2½ tablespoons Tahini (see here)
- 2½ tablespoons Maple syrup
- 2 teaspoons Vanilla extract
- ⅔ cup Vegan semisweet or bittersweet chocolate chips
- Baking spray

Directions:

1. Preheat the air fryer to 325°F (or 330°F, if that's the closest setting).

2. Whisk the flour, oats, baking soda, and salt in a bowl until well combined.

3. Using an electric hand mixer at medium speed, beat the sugar, oil, tahini, maple syrup, and vanilla until rich and creamy, about 3 minutes, scraping down the inside of the bowl occasionally.

4. Scrape down and remove the beaters. Fold in the flour mixture and chocolate chips with a rubber spatula just until all the flour is moistened and the chocolate chips are even throughout the dough.

5. For a small air fryer, coat the inside of a 6-inch round cake pan with baking spray. For a medium air fryer, coat the inside of a 7-inch round cake pan with baking spray. And for a large air fryer, coat the inside of an 8-inch round cake pan with baking spray. Scrape and gently press the dough into the prepared pan, spreading it into an even layer to the perimeter.

6. Set the pan in the basket and air-fry undisturbed for 16 minutes, or until puffed, browned, and firm to the touch.

7. Transfer the pan to a wire rack and cool for 10 minutes. Loosen the cookie from the perimeter with a spatula, then invert the pan onto a cutting board and let the cookie come free. Remove the pan and reinvert the cookie onto the wire rack. Cool for 5 minutes more before slicing into wedges to serve.

Chewy Coconut Cake

Servings: 6
Cooking Time: 18-22 Minutes

Ingredients:

- ¾ cup plus 2½ tablespoons All-purpose flour
- ¾ teaspoon Baking powder
- ⅛ teaspoon Table salt
- 7½ tablespoons (1 stick minus ½ tablespoon) Butter, at room temperature
- ⅓ cup plus 1 tablespoon Granulated white sugar
- 5 tablespoons Packed light brown sugar
- 5 tablespoons Pasteurized egg substitute, such as Egg Beaters
- 2 teaspoons Vanilla extract
- ½ cup Unsweetened shredded coconut (see here)
- Baking spray

Directions:

1. Preheat the air fryer to 325°F (or 330°F, if that's the closest setting).

2. Mix the flour, baking powder, and salt in a small bowl until well combined.

3. Using an electric hand mixer at medium speed , beat the butter, granulated white sugar, and brown sugar in a medium bowl until creamy and smooth, about 3 minutes, occasionally scraping down the inside of the bowl. Beat in the egg substitute or egg and vanilla until smooth.

4. Scrape down and remove the beaters. Fold in the flour mixture with a rubber spatula just until all the flour is moistened. Fold in the coconut until the mixture is a uniform color.

5. Use the baking spray to generously coat the inside of a 6-inch round cake pan for a small batch, a 7-inch round cake pan for a medium batch, or an 8-inch round cake pan for a large batch. Scrape and spread the batter into the pan, smoothing the batter out to an even layer.

6. Set the pan in the basket and air-fry for 18 minutes for a 6-inch layer, 20 minutes for a 7-inch layer, or 22 minutes for an 8-inch layer, or until the cake is well browned and set even if there's a little soft give right at the center. Start checking it at the 16-minute mark to know where you are.

7. Use hot pads or silicone baking mitts to transfer the cake pan to a wire rack. Cool for at least 1 hour or up to 4 hours. Use a nonstick-safe knife to slice the cake into wedges right in the pan, lifting them out one by one.

White Chocolate Cranberry Blondies

Servings: 6
Cooking Time: 18 Minutes

Ingredients:

- ⅓ cup butter
- ½ cup sugar
- 1 teaspoon vanilla extract
- 1 large egg
- 1 cup all-purpose flour
- ½ teaspoon baking powder
- ⅛ teaspoon salt
- ¼ cup dried cranberries
- ¼ cup white chocolate chips

Directions:

1. Preheat the air fryer to 320°F.

2. In a large bowl, cream the butter with the sugar and vanilla extract. Whisk in the egg and set aside.

3. In a separate bowl, mix the flour with the baking powder and salt. Then gently mix the dry ingredients into the wet. Fold in the cranberries and chocolate chips.

4. Liberally spray an oven-safe 7-inch springform pan with olive oil and pour the batter into the pan.

5. Cook for 17 minutes or until a toothpick inserted in the center comes out clean.

6. Remove and let cool 5 minutes before serving.

Baked Apple

Servings: 6

Cooking Time: 20 Minutes

Ingredients:

- 3 small Honey Crisp or other baking apples
- 3 tablespoons maple syrup
- 3 tablespoons chopped pecans
- 1 tablespoon firm butter, cut into 6 pieces

Directions:

1. Put ½ cup water in the drawer of the air fryer.

2. Wash apples well and dry them.

3. Split apples in half. Remove core and a little of the flesh to make a cavity for the pecans.

4. Place apple halves in air fryer basket, cut side up.

5. Spoon 1½ teaspoons pecans into each cavity.

6. Spoon ½ tablespoon maple syrup over pecans in each apple.

7. Top each apple with ½ teaspoon butter.

8. Cook at 360°F for 20 minutes, until apples are tender.

Bananas Foster Bread Pudding

Servings: 4

Cooking Time: 25 Minutes

Ingredients:

- ½ cup brown sugar
- 3 eggs
- ¾ cup half and half
- 1 teaspoon pure vanilla extract
- 6 cups cubed Kings Hawaiian bread (½-inch cubes), ½ pound
- 2 bananas, sliced
- 1 cup caramel sauce, plus more for serving

Directions:

1. Preheat the air fryer to 350°F.

2. Combine the brown sugar, eggs, half and half and vanilla extract in a large bowl, whisking until the sugar has dissolved and the mixture is smooth. Stir in the cubed bread and toss to coat all the cubes evenly. Let the bread sit for 10 minutes to absorb the liquid.

3. Mix the sliced bananas and caramel sauce together in a separate bowl.

4. Fill the bottom of 4 (8-ounce) greased ramekins with half the bread cubes. Divide the caramel and bananas between the ramekins, spooning them on top of the bread cubes. Top with the remaining bread cubes and wrap each ramekin with aluminum foil, tenting the foil at the top to leave some room for the bread to puff up during the cooking process.

5. Air-fry two bread puddings at a time for 25 minutes. Let the puddings cool a little and serve warm with additional caramel sauce drizzled on top. A scoop of vanilla ice cream would be nice too and in keeping with our Bananas Foster theme!

Vanilla Butter Cake

Servings: 6

Cooking Time: 20-24 Minutes

Ingredients:

- ¾ cup plus 1 tablespoon All-purpose flour
- 1 teaspoon Baking powder
- ¼ teaspoon Table salt
- 8 tablespoons (½ cup/1 stick) Butter, at room temperature
- ½ cup Granulated white sugar
- 2 Large egg(s)
- 2 tablespoons Whole or low-fat milk (not fat-free)
- ¾ teaspoon Vanilla extract
- Baking spray (see here)

Directions:

1. Preheat the air fryer to 325°F (or 330°F, if that's the closest setting).

2. Mix the flour, baking powder, and salt in a small bowl until well combined.

3. Using an electric hand mixer at medium speed, beat the butter and sugar in a medium bowl until creamy and smooth, about 3 minutes, occasionally scraping down the inside of the bowl.

4. Beat in the egg or eggs, as well as the white or a yolk as necessary. Beat in the milk and vanilla until smooth. Turn off the beaters and add the flour mixture. Beat at low speed until thick and smooth.

5. Use the baking spray to generously coat the inside of a 6-inch round cake pan for a small batch, a 7-inch round cake pan for a medium batch, or an 8-inch round cake pan for a large batch. Scrape and spread the batter into the pan, smoothing the batter out to an even layer.

6. Set the pan in the basket and air-fry undisturbed for 20 minutes for a 6-inch layer, 22 minutes for a 7-inch layer, or 24 minutes for an 8-inch layer, or until a toothpick or cake tester inserted into the center of the cake comes out clean. Start checking it at the 15-minute mark to know where you are.

7. Use hot pads or silicone baking mitts to transfer the cake pan to a wire rack. Cool for 5 minutes. To unmold, set a cutting board over the baking pan and invert both the board and the pan. Lift the still-warm pan off the cake layer. Set the wire rack on top of the cake layer and invert all of it with the cutting board so that the cake layer is now right side up on the wire rack. Remove the cutting board and continue cooling the cake for at least 10 minutes or to room temperature, about 30 minutes, before slicing into wedges.

Almond-roasted Pears

Servings: 4

Cooking Time: 15 Minutes

Ingredients:

- Yogurt Topping
- 1 container vanilla Greek yogurt (5–6 ounces)
- ¼ teaspoon almond flavoring
- 2 whole pears
- ¼ cup crushed Biscoff cookies (approx. 4 cookies)
- 1 tablespoon sliced almonds
- 1 tablespoon butter

Directions:

1. Stir almond flavoring into yogurt and set aside while preparing pears.

2. Halve each pear and spoon out the core.

3. Place pear halves in air fryer basket.

4. Stir together the cookie crumbs and almonds. Place a quarter of this mixture into the hollow of each pear half.

5. Cut butter into 4 pieces and place one piece on top of crumb mixture in each pear.

6. Cook at 360°F for 15 minutes or until pears have cooked through but are still slightly firm.

7. Serve pears warm with a dollop of yogurt topping.

Honey-roasted Mixed Nuts

Servings: 8

Cooking Time: 15 Minutes

Ingredients:

- ½ cup raw, shelled pistachios
- ½ cup raw almonds
- 1 cup raw walnuts
- 2 tablespoons filtered water
- 2 tablespoons honey
- 1 tablespoon vegetable oil
- 2 tablespoons sugar
- ½ teaspoon salt

Directions:

1. Preheat the air fryer to 300°F.

2. Lightly spray an air-fryer-safe pan with olive oil; then place the pistachios, almonds, and walnuts inside the pan and place the pan inside the air fryer basket.

3. Cook for 15 minutes, shaking the basket every 5 minutes to rotate the nuts.

4. While the nuts are roasting, boil the water in a small pan and stir in the honey and oil. Continue to stir while cooking until the water begins to evaporate and a thick sauce is formed. Note: The sauce should stick to the back of a wooden spoon when mixed. Turn off the heat.

5. Remove the nuts from the air fryer (cooking should have just completed) and spoon the nuts into the stovetop pan. Use a spatula to coat the nuts with the honey syrup.

6. Line a baking sheet with parchment paper and spoon the nuts onto the sheet. Lightly sprinkle the sugar and salt over the nuts and let cool in the refrigerator for at least 2 hours.

7. When the honey and sugar have hardened, store the nuts in an airtight container in the refrigerator.

Thumbprint Sugar Cookies

Servings: 10

Cooking Time: 8 Minutes

Ingredients:

- 2½ tablespoons butter
- ⅓ cup cane sugar
- 1 teaspoon pure vanilla extract
- 1 large egg
- 1 cup all-purpose flour
- ½ teaspoon baking soda
- ¼ teaspoon salt
- 10 chocolate kisses

Directions:

1. Preheat the air fryer to 350°F.

2. In a large bowl, cream the butter with the sugar and vanilla. Whisk in the egg and set aside.

3. In a separate bowl, mix the flour, baking soda, and salt. Then gently mix the dry ingredients into the wet. Portion the dough into 10 balls; then press down on each with the bottom of a cup to create a flat cookie.

4. Liberally spray the metal trivet of an air fryer basket with olive oil mist.

5. Place the cookies in the air fryer basket on the trivet and cook for 8 minutes or until the tops begin to lightly brown.

6. Remove and immediately press the chocolate kisses into the tops of the cookies while still warm.

7. Let cool 5 minutes and then enjoy.

Nutella® Torte

Servings: 6

Cooking Time: 55 Minutes

Ingredients:

- ¼ cup unsalted butter, softened
- ½ cup sugar
- 2 eggs
- 1 teaspoon vanilla
- 1¼ cups Nutella® (or other chocolate hazelnut spread), divided
- ¼ cup flour
- 1 teaspoon baking powder
- ¼ teaspoon salt
- dark chocolate fudge topping
- coarsely chopped toasted hazelnuts

Directions:

1. Cream the butter and sugar together with an electric hand mixer until light and fluffy. Add the eggs, vanilla, and ¾ cup of the Nutella® and mix until combined. Combine the flour, baking powder and salt together, and add these dry ingredients to the butter mixture, beating for 1 minute.

2. Preheat the air fryer to 350°F.

3. Grease a 7-inch cake pan with butter and then line the bottom of the pan with a circle of parchment paper. Grease the parchment paper circle as well. Pour the batter into the prepared cake pan and wrap the pan completely with aluminum foil. Lower the pan into the air fryer basket with an aluminum sling (fold a piece of aluminum foil into a strip about 2-inches wide by 24-inches long). Fold the ends of the aluminum foil over the top of the dish before returning the basket to the air fryer. Air-fry for 30 minutes. Remove the foil and air-fry for another 25 minutes.

4. Remove the cake from air fryer and let it cool for 10 minutes. Invert the cake onto a plate, remove the parchment paper and invert the cake back onto a serving platter. While the cake is still warm, spread the remaining ½ cup of Nutella® over the top of the cake. Melt the dark chocolate fudge in the microwave for about 10 seconds so it melts enough to be pourable. Drizzle the sauce on top of the cake in a zigzag motion. Turn the cake 90 degrees and drizzle more sauce in zigzags perpendicular to the first zigzags. Garnish the edges of the torte with the toasted hazelnuts and serve.

S'mores Pockets

Servings: 6

Cooking Time: 5 Minutes

Ingredients:

- 12 sheets phyllo dough, thawed
- 1½ cups butter, melted
- ¾ cup graham cracker crumbs
- 1 (7-ounce) Giant Hershey's® milk chocolate bar
- 12 marshmallows, cut in half

Directions:

1. Place one sheet of the phyllo on a large cutting board. Keep the rest of the phyllo sheets covered with a slightly damp, clean kitchen towel. Brush the phyllo sheet generously with some melted butter. Place a second phyllo sheet on top of the first and brush it with more butter. Repeat with one more phyllo sheet until you have a stack of 3 phyllo sheets with butter brushed between the layers. Cover the phyllo sheets with one quarter of the graham cracker crumbs leaving a 1-inch border on one of the short ends of the rectangle. Cut the phyllo sheets lengthwise into 3 strips.

2. Take 2 of the strips and crisscross them to form a cross with the empty borders at the top and to the left. Place 2 of the chocolate rectangles in the center of the cross. Place 4 of the marshmallow halves on top of the chocolate. Now fold the pocket together by folding the bottom phyllo strip up over the chocolate and marshmallows. Then fold the right side over, then the top strip down and finally the left side over. Brush all the edges generously with melted butter to seal shut. Repeat with the next three sheets of phyllo, until all the sheets have been used. You will be able to make 2 pockets with every second batch because you will have an extra graham cracker crumb strip from the previous set of sheets.

3. Preheat the air fryer to 350°F.

4. Transfer 3 pockets at a time to the air fryer basket. Air-fry at 350°F for 4 to 5 minutes, until the phyllo dough is light brown in color. Flip the pockets over halfway through the cooking process. Repeat with the remaining 3 pockets.

5. Serve warm.

Annie's Chocolate Chunk Hazelnut Cookies

Servings: 24

Cooking Time: 12 Minutes

Ingredients:

- 1 cup butter, softened
- 1 cup brown sugar
- ½ cup granulated sugar
- 2 eggs, lightly beaten
- 1½ teaspoons vanilla extract
- 1½ cups all-purpose flour
- ½ cup rolled oats
- 1 teaspoon baking soda
- ½ teaspoon salt
- 2 cups chocolate chunks
- ½ cup toasted chopped hazelnuts

Directions:

1. Cream the butter and sugars together until light and fluffy using a stand mixer or electric hand mixer. Add the eggs and vanilla, and beat until well combined.

2. Combine the flour, rolled oats, baking soda and salt in a second bowl. Gradually add the dry ingredients to the wet ingredients with a wooden spoon or spatula. Stir in the chocolate chunks and hazelnuts until distributed throughout the dough.

3. Shape the cookies into small balls about the size of golf balls and place them on a baking sheet. Freeze the cookie balls for at least 30 minutes, or package them in as airtight a package as you can and keep them in your freezer.

4. When you're ready for a delicious snack or dessert, Preheat the air fryer to 350°F. Cut a piece of parchment paper to fit the number of cookies you are baking. Place the parchment down in the air fryer basket and place the frozen cookie ball or balls on top (remember to leave room for them to expand).

5. Air-fry the cookies at 350°F for 12 minutes, or until they are done to your liking. Let them cool for a few minutes before enjoying your freshly baked cookie.

Cheese Blintzes

Servings: 6

Cooking Time: 10 Minutes

Ingredients:

- 1½ 7½-ounce package(s) farmer cheese
- 3 tablespoons Regular or low-fat cream cheese (not fat-free)
- 3 tablespoons Granulated white sugar
- ¼ teaspoon Vanilla extract
- 6 Egg roll wrappers
- 3 tablespoons Butter, melted and cooled

Directions:

1. Preheat the air fryer to 375°F .

2. Use a flatware fork to mash the farmer cheese, cream cheese, sugar, and vanilla in a small bowl until smooth.

3. Set one egg roll wrapper on a clean, dry work surface. Place ¼ cup of the filling at the edge closest to you, leaving a ½-inch gap before the edge of the wrapper. Dip your clean finger in water and wet the edges of the wrapper. Fold the perpendicular sides over the filling, then roll the wrapper closed with the filling inside. Set it aside seam side down and continue filling the remainder of the wrappers.

4. Brush the wrappers on all sides with the melted butter. Be generous. Set them seam side down in the basket with as much space between them as possible. Air-fry undisturbed for 10 minutes, or until lightly browned.

5. Use a nonstick-safe spatula to transfer the blintzes to a wire rack. Cool for at least 5 minutes or up to 20 minutes before serving.

Giant Buttery Oatmeal Cookie

Servings: 4

Cooking Time: 16 Minutes

Ingredients:

- 1 cup Rolled oats (not quick-cooking or steel-cut oats)
- ½ cup All-purpose flour
- ½ teaspoon Baking soda
- ½ teaspoon Ground cinnamon
- ½ teaspoon Table salt
- 3½ tablespoons Butter, at room temperature
- ⅓ cup Packed dark brown sugar
- 1½ tablespoons Granulated white sugar
- 3 tablespoons (or 1 medium egg, well beaten) Pasteurized egg substitute, such as Egg Beaters
- ¾ teaspoon Vanilla extract
- ⅓ cup Chopped pecans
- Baking spray

Directions:

1. Preheat the air fryer to 350°F .

2. Stir the oats, flour, baking soda, cinnamon, and salt in a bowl until well combined.

3. Using an electric hand mixer at medium speed , beat the butter, brown sugar, and granulated white sugar until creamy and thick, about 3 minutes, scraping down the inside of the bowl occasionally. Beat in the egg substitute or egg (as applicable) and vanilla until uniform.

4. Scrape down and remove the beaters. Fold in the flour mixture and pecans with a rubber spatula just until all the flour is moistened and the nuts are even throughout the dough.

5. For a small air fryer, coat the inside of a 6-inch round cake pan with baking spray. For a medium air fryer, coat the inside of a 7-inch round cake pan with baking spray. And for a large air fryer, coat the inside of an 8-inch round cake pan with baking spray. Scrape and gently press the dough into the prepared pan, spreading it into an even layer to the perimeter.

6. Set the pan in the basket and air-fry undisturbed for 16 minutes, or until puffed and browned.

7. Transfer the pan to a wire rack and cool for 10 minutes. Loosen the cookie from the perimeter with a spatula, then invert the pan onto a cutting board and let the cookie come free. Remove the pan and reinvert the cookie onto the wire rack. Cool for 5 minutes more before slicing into wedges to serve.

Keto Cheesecake Cups

Servings: 6
Cooking Time: 10 Minutes
Ingredients:
- 8 ounces cream cheese
- ¼ cup plain whole-milk Greek yogurt
- 1 large egg
- 1 teaspoon pure vanilla extract
- 3 tablespoons monk fruit sweetener
- ¼ teaspoon salt
- ½ cup walnuts, roughly chopped

Directions:
1. Preheat the air fryer to 315°F.
2. In a large bowl, use a hand mixer to beat the cream cheese together with the yogurt, egg, vanilla, sweetener, and salt. When combined, fold in the chopped walnuts.
3. Set 6 silicone muffin liners inside an air-fryer-safe pan. Note: This is to allow for an easier time getting the cheesecake bites in and out. If you don't have a pan, you can place them directly in the air fryer basket.
4. Evenly fill the cupcake liners with cheesecake batter.
5. Carefully place the pan into the air fryer basket and cook for about 10 minutes, or until the tops are lightly browned and firm.

6. Carefully remove the pan when done and place in the refrigerator for 3 hours to firm up before serving.

Easy Churros

Servings: 12
Cooking Time: 10 Minutes
Ingredients:
- ½ cup Water
- 4 tablespoons (¼ cup/½ stick) Butter
- ¼ teaspoon Table salt
- ½ cup All-purpose flour
- 2 Large egg(s)
- ¼ cup Granulated white sugar
- 2 teaspoons Ground cinnamon

Directions:
1. Bring the water, butter, and salt to a boil in a small saucepan set over high heat, stirring occasionally.
2. When the butter has fully melted, reduce the heat to medium and stir in the flour to form a dough. Continue cooking, stirring constantly, to dry out the dough until it coats the bottom and sides of the pan with a film, even a crust. Remove the pan from the heat, scrape the dough into a bowl, and cool for 15 minutes.
3. Using an electric hand mixer at medium speed, beat in the egg, or eggs one at a time, until the dough is smooth and firm enough to hold its shape.
4. Mix the sugar and cinnamon in a small bowl. Scoop up 1 tablespoon of the dough and roll it in the sugar mixture to form a small, coated tube about ½ inch in diameter and 2 inches long. Set it aside and make 5 more tubes for the small batch or 11 more for the large one.

5. Set the tubes on a plate and freeze for 20 minutes. Meanwhile, Preheat the air fryer to 375°F .

6. Set 3 frozen tubes in the basket for a small batch or 6 for a large one with as much air space between them as possible. Air-fry undisturbed for 10 minutes, or until puffed, brown, and set.

7. Use kitchen tongs to transfer the churros to a wire rack to cool for at least 5 minutes. Meanwhile, air-fry and cool the second batch of churros in the same way.

Cheesecake Wontons

Servings:16

Cooking Time: 6 Minutes

Ingredients:

- ¼ cup Regular or low-fat cream cheese (not fat-free)
- 2 tablespoons Granulated white sugar
- 1½ tablespoons Egg yolk
- ¼ teaspoon Vanilla extract
- ⅛ teaspoon Table salt
- 1½ tablespoons All-purpose flour
- 16 Wonton wrappers (vegetarian, if a concern)
- Vegetable oil spray

Directions:

1. Preheat the air fryer to 400°F.

2. Using a flatware fork, mash the cream cheese, sugar, egg yolk, and vanilla in a small bowl until smooth. Add the salt and flour and continue mashing until evenly combined.

3. Set a wonton wrapper on a clean, dry work surface so that one corner faces you (so that it looks like a diamond on your work surface). Set 1 teaspoon of the cream cheese mixture in the middle of the wrapper but just above a horizontal line that would divide the wrapper in half. Dip your clean finger in water and run it along the edges of the wrapper. Fold the corner closest to you up and over the filling, lining it up with the corner farthest from you, thereby making a stuffed triangle. Press gently to seal. Wet the two triangle tips nearest you, then fold them up and together over the filling. Gently press together to seal and fuse. Set aside and continue making more stuffed wontons, 11 more for the small batch, 15 more for the medium batch, or 23 more for the large one.

4. Lightly coat the stuffed wrappers on all sides with vegetable oil spray. Set them with the fused corners up in the basket with as much air space between them as possible. Air-fry undisturbed for 6 minutes, or until golden brown and crisp.

5. Gently dump the contents of the basket onto a wire rack. Cool for at least 5 minutes before serving.

Custard

Servings: 4

Cooking Time: 45 Minutes

Ingredients:

- 2 cups whole milk
- 2 eggs
- ¼ cup sugar
- ⅛ teaspoon salt
- ¼ teaspoon vanilla
- cooking spray
- ⅛ teaspoon nutmeg

Directions:

1. In a blender, process milk, egg, sugar, salt, and vanilla until smooth.

2. Spray a 6 x 6-inch baking pan with nonstick spray and pour the custard into it.

3. Cook at 300°F for 45 minutes. Custard is done when the center sets.

4. Sprinkle top with the nutmeg.

5. Allow custard to cool slightly.

6. Serve it warm, at room temperature, or chilled.

Honey-pecan Yogurt Cake

Servings: 6
Cooking Time: 18-24 Minutes
Ingredients:

- 1 cup plus 3½ tablespoons All-purpose flour
- ¼ teaspoon Baking powder
- ¼ teaspoon Baking soda
- ¼ teaspoon Table salt
- 5 tablespoons Plain full-fat, low-fat, or fat-free Greek yogurt
- 5 tablespoons Honey
- 5 tablespoons Pasteurized egg substitute, such as Egg Beaters
- 2 teaspoons Vanilla extract
- ⅔ cup Chopped pecans
- Baking spray (see here)

Directions:

1. Preheat the air fryer to 325°F (or 330°F, if the closest setting).

2. Mix the flour, baking powder, baking soda, and salt in a small bowl until well combined.

3. Using an electric hand mixer at medium speed , beat the yogurt, honey, egg substitute or egg, and vanilla in a medium bowl until smooth, about 2 minutes, scraping down the inside of the bowl once or twice.

4. Turn off the mixer; scrape down and remove the beaters. Fold in the flour mixture with a rubber spatula, just until all of the flour has been moistened. Fold in the pecans until they are evenly distributed in the mixture.

5. Use the baking spray to generously coat the inside of a 6-inch round cake pan for a small batch, a 7-inch round cake pan for a medium batch, or an 8-inch round cake pan for a large batch. Scrape and spread the batter into the pan, smoothing the batter out to an even layer.

6. Set the pan in the basket and air-fry for 18 minutes for a 6-inch layer, 22 minutes for a 7-inch layer, or 24 minutes for an 8-inch layer, or until a toothpick or cake tester inserted into the center of the cake comes out clean. Start checking it at the 15-minute mark to know where you are.

7. Use hot pads or silicone baking mitts to transfer the cake pan to a wire rack. Cool for 5 minutes. To unmold, set a cutting board over the baking pan and invert both the board and the pan. Lift the still-warm pan off the cake layer. Set the wire rack on top of that layer and invert all of it with the cutting board so that the cake layer is now right side up on the wire rack. Remove the cutting board and continue cooling the cake for at least 10 minutes or to room temperature, about 30 minutes, before slicing into wedges.

Blueberry Crisp

Servings: 6
Cooking Time: 13 Minutes
Ingredients:

- 3 cups Fresh or thawed frozen blueberries
- ⅓ cup Granulated white sugar
- 1 tablespoon Instant tapioca
- ⅓ cup All-purpose flour
- ⅓ cup Rolled oats (not quick-cooking or steel-cut)
- ⅓ cup Chopped walnuts or pecans
- ⅓ cup Packed light brown sugar
- 5 tablespoons plus 1 teaspoon (⅔ stick) Butter, melted and cooled
- ¾ teaspoon Ground cinnamon
- ¼ teaspoon Table salt

Directions:

1. Preheat the air fryer to 400°F.

2. Mix the blueberries, granulated white sugar, and instant tapioca in a 6-inch round cake pan for a small batch, a 7-inch round cake pan for a medium batch, or an 8-inch round cake pan for a large batch.

3. When the machine is at temperature, set the cake pan in the basket and air-fry undisturbed for 5 minutes, or just until the blueberries begin to bubble.

4. Meanwhile, mix the flour, oats, nuts, brown sugar, butter, cinnamon, and salt in a medium bowl until well combined.

5. When the blueberries have begun to bubble, crumble this flour mixture evenly on top. Continue air-frying undisturbed for 8 minutes, or until the topping has browned a bit and the filling is bubbling.

6. Use two hot pads or silicone baking mitts to transfer the cake pan to a wire rack. Cool for at least 10 minutes or to room temperature before serving.

Roasted Pears

Servings: 4
Cooking Time: 10 Minutes
Ingredients:
- 2 Ripe pears, preferably Anjou, stemmed, peeled, halved lengthwise, and cored
- 2 tablespoons Butter, melted
- 2 teaspoons Granulated white sugar
- Grated nutmeg
- ¼ cup Honey
- ½ cup (about 1½ ounces) Shaved Parmesan cheese

Directions:
1. Preheat the air fryer to 400°F.
2. Brush each pear half with about 1½ teaspoons of the melted butter, then sprinkle their cut sides with ½ teaspoon sugar. Grate a pinch of nutmeg over each pear.

3. When the machine is at temperature, set the pear halves cut side up in the basket with as much air space between them as possible. Air-fry undisturbed for 10 minutes, or until hot and softened.

4. Use a nonstick-safe spatula, and perhaps a flatware tablespoon for balance, to transfer the pear halves to a serving platter or plates. Cool for a minute or two, then drizzle each pear half with 1 tablespoon of the honey. Lay about 2 tablespoons of shaved Parmesan over each half just before serving.

Fried Oreos

Servings: 12
Cooking Time: 6 Minutes Per Batch
Ingredients:
- oil for misting or nonstick spray
- 1 cup complete pancake and waffle mix
- 1 teaspoon vanilla extract
- ½ cup water, plus 2 tablespoons
- 12 Oreos or other chocolate sandwich cookies
- 1 tablespoon confectioners' sugar

Directions:
1. Spray baking pan with oil or nonstick spray and place in basket.
2. Preheat air fryer to 390°F.
3. In a medium bowl, mix together the pancake mix, vanilla, and water.
4. Dip 4 cookies in batter and place in baking pan.
5. Cook for 6minutes, until browned.
6. Repeat steps 4 and 5 for the remaining cookies.
7. Sift sugar over warm cookies.

Fried Snickers Bars

Servings:8

Cooking Time: 4 Minutes

Ingredients:

- ⅓ cup All-purpose flour
- 1 Large egg white(s), beaten until foamy
- 1½ cups (6 ounces) Vanilla wafer cookie crumbs
- 8 Fun-size (0.6-ounce/17-gram) Snickers bars, frozen
- Vegetable oil spray

Directions:

1. Preheat the air fryer to 400°F.

2. Set up and fill three shallow soup plates or small pie plates on your counter: one for the flour, one for the beaten egg white(s), and one for the cookie crumbs.

3. Unwrap the frozen candy bars. Dip one in the flour, turning it to coat on all sides. Gently shake off any excess, then set it in the beaten egg white(s). Turn it to coat all sides, even the ends, then let any excess egg white slip back into the rest. Set the candy bar in the cookie crumbs. Turn to coat on all sides, even the ends. Dip the candy bar back in the egg white(s) a second time, then into the cookie crumbs a second time, making sure you have an even coating all around. Coat the covered candy bar all over with vegetable oil spray. Set aside so you can dip and coat the remaining candy bars.

4. Set the coated candy bars in the basket with as much air space between them as possible. Air-fry undisturbed for 4 minutes, or until golden brown.

5. Remove the basket from the machine and let the candy bars cool in the basket for 10 minutes. Use a nonstick-safe spatula to transfer them to a wire rack and cool for 5 minutes more before chowing down.

Giant Oatmeal–peanut Butter Cookie

Servings: 4

Cooking Time: 18 Minutes

Ingredients:

- 1 cup Rolled oats (not quick-cooking or steel-cut oats)
- ½ cup All-purpose flour
- ½ teaspoon Ground cinnamon
- ½ teaspoon Baking soda
- ⅓ cup Packed light brown sugar
- ¼ cup Solid vegetable shortening
- 2 tablespoons Natural-style creamy peanut butter
- 3 tablespoons Granulated white sugar
- 2 tablespoons (or 1 small egg, well beaten) Pasteurized egg substitute, such as Egg Beaters
- ⅓ cup Roasted, salted peanuts, chopped
- Baking spray

Directions:

1. Preheat the air fryer to 350°F .

2. Stir the oats, flour, cinnamon, and baking soda in a bowl until well combined.

3. Using an electric hand mixer at medium speed, beat the brown sugar, shortening, peanut butter, granulated white sugar, and egg substitute or egg (as applicable) until smooth and creamy, about 3 minutes, scraping down the inside of the bowl occasionally.

4. Scrape down and remove the beaters. Fold in the flour mixture and peanuts with a rubber spatula just until all the flour is moistened and the peanut bits are evenly distributed in the dough.

5. For a small air fryer, coat the inside of a 6-inch round cake pan with baking spray. For a medium air fryer, coat the inside of a 7-inch round cake pan with baking spray. And for a large air fryer, coat the inside of an 8-inch round cake pan with baking spray. Scrape and gently press the dough into the prepared pan, spreading it into an even layer to the perimeter.

6. Set the pan in the basket and air-fry undisturbed for 18 minutes, or until well browned.

7. Transfer the pan to a wire rack and cool for 15 minutes. Loosen the cookie from the perimeter with a spatula, then invert the pan onto a cutting board and let the cookie come free. Remove the pan and reinvert the cookie onto the wire rack. Cool for 5 minutes more before slicing into wedges to serve.

Blueberry Cheesecake Tartlets

Servings: 9
Cooking Time: 6 Minutes

Ingredients:

- 8 ounces cream cheese, softened
- ¼ cup sugar
- 1 egg
- ½ teaspoon vanilla extract
- zest of 2 lemons, divided
- 9 mini graham cracker tartlet shells*
- 2 cups blueberries
- ½ teaspoon ground cinnamon
- juice of ½ lemon
- ¼ cup apricot preserves

Directions:

1. Preheat the air fryer to 330°F.

2. Combine the cream cheese, sugar, egg, vanilla and the zest of one lemon in a medium bowl and blend until smooth by hand or with an electric hand mixer. Pour the cream cheese mixture into the tartlet shells.

3. Air-fry 3 tartlets at a time at 330°F for 6 minutes, rotating them in the air fryer basket halfway through the cooking time.

4. Combine the blueberries, cinnamon, zest of one lemon and juice of half a lemon in a bowl. Melt the apricot preserves in the microwave or over low heat in a saucepan. Pour the apricot preserves over the blueberries and gently toss to coat.

5. Allow the cheesecakes to cool completely and then top each one with some of the blueberry mixture. Garnish the tartlets with a little sugared lemon peel and refrigerate until you are ready to serve.

Chocolate Soufflés

Servings: 2
Cooking Time: 14 Minutes

Ingredients:

- butter and sugar for greasing the ramekins
- 3 ounces semi-sweet chocolate, chopped
- ¼ cup unsalted butter
- 2 eggs, yolks and white separated
- 3 tablespoons sugar
- ½ teaspoon pure vanilla extract
- 2 tablespoons all-purpose flour
- powdered sugar, for dusting the finished soufflés
- heavy cream, for serving

Directions:

1. Butter and sugar two 6-ounce ramekins. (Butter the ramekins and then coat the butter with sugar by shaking it around in the ramekin and dumping out any excess.)

2. Melt the chocolate and butter together, either in the microwave or in a double boiler. In a

separate bowl, beat the egg yolks vigorously. Add the sugar and the vanilla extract and beat well again. Drizzle in the chocolate and butter, mixing well. Stir in the flour, combining until there are no lumps.

3. Preheat the air fryer to 330°F.

4. In a separate bowl, whisk the egg whites to soft peak stage (the point at which the whites can almost stand up on the end of your whisk). Fold the whipped egg whites into the chocolate mixture gently and in stages.

5. Transfer the batter carefully to the buttered ramekins, leaving about ½-inch at the top. (You may have a little extra batter, depending on how airy the batter is, so you might be able to squeeze out a third soufflé if you want to.) Place the ramekins into the air fryer basket and air-fry for 14 minutes. The soufflés should have risen nicely and be brown on top. (Don't worry if the top gets a little dark – you'll be covering it with powdered sugar in the next step.)

6. Dust with powdered sugar and serve immediately with heavy cream to pour over the top at the table.

Spaghetti Squash And Kale Fritters With Pomodoro Sauce

Servings: 3
Cooking Time: 45 Minutes
Ingredients:
- 1½-pound spaghetti squash (about half a large or a whole small squash)
- olive oil
- ½ onion, diced
- ½ red bell pepper, diced
- 2 cloves garlic, minced
- 4 cups coarsely chopped kale
- salt and freshly ground black pepper
- 1 egg
- ⅓ cup breadcrumbs, divided*
- ⅓ cup grated Parmesan cheese
- ½ teaspoon dried rubbed sage
- pinch nutmeg
- Pomodoro Sauce:
- 2 tablespoons olive oil
- ½ onion, chopped
- 1 to 2 cloves garlic, minced
- 1 (28-ounce) can peeled tomatoes
- ¼ cup red wine
- 1 teaspoon Italian seasoning
- 2 tablespoons chopped fresh basil, plus more for garnish
- salt and freshly ground black pepper
- ½ teaspoon sugar (optional)

Directions:
1. Preheat the air fryer to 370°F.
2. Cut the spaghetti squash in half lengthwise and remove the seeds. Rub the inside of the squash with olive oil and season with salt and pepper. Place the squash, cut side up, into the air fryer basket and air-fry for 30 minutes, flipping the squash over halfway through the cooking process.
3. While the squash is cooking, Preheat a large sauté pan over medium heat on the stovetop. Add a little olive oil and sauté the onions for 3 minutes, until they start to soften. Add the red pepper and garlic and continue to sauté for an additional 4 minutes. Add the kale and season with salt and pepper. Cook for 2 more minutes, or until the kale is soft. Transfer the mixture to a large bowl and let it cool.
4. While the squash continues to cook, make the Pomodoro sauce. Preheat the large sauté pan again over medium heat on the stovetop. Add the olive oil and sauté the onion and garlic for 2 to 3 minutes, until the onion begins to soften. Crush the canned tomatoes with your hands and add them to the pan along with the red wine and Italian seasoning and simmer for 20 minutes. Add the basil and season to taste with salt, pepper and sugar (if using).
5. When the spaghetti squash has finished cooking, use a fork to scrape the inside flesh of the squash onto a sheet pan. Spread the squash out and let it cool.
6. Once cool, add the spaghetti squash to the kale mixture, along with the egg, breadcrumbs, Parmesan cheese, sage, nutmeg, salt and freshly ground black pepper. Stir to combine well and then divide the mixture into 6 thick portions. You can shape the portions into patties, but I prefer to keep them a little random and unique in shape. Spray or brush the fritters with olive oil.
7. Preheat the air fryer to 370°F.

8. Brush the air fryer basket with a little olive oil and transfer the fritters to the basket. Air-fry the squash and kale fritters at 370°F for 15 minutes, flipping them over halfway through the cooking process.

9. Serve the fritters warm with the Pomodoro sauce spooned over the top or pooled on your plate. Garnish with the fresh basil leaves.

Curried Potato, Cauliflower And Pea Turnovers

Servings: 4

Cooking Time: 40 Minutes

Ingredients:

- Dough:
- 2 cups all-purpose flour
- ½ teaspoon baking powder
- 1 teaspoon salt
- freshly ground black pepper
- ¼ teaspoon dried thyme
- ¼ cup canola oil
- ½ to ⅔ cup water
- Turnover Filling:
- 1 tablespoon canola or vegetable oil
- 1 onion, finely chopped
- 1 clove garlic, minced
- 1 tablespoon grated fresh ginger
- ½ teaspoon cumin seeds
- ½ teaspoon fennel seeds
- 1 teaspoon curry powder
- 2 russet potatoes, diced
- 2 cups cauliflower florets
- ½ cup frozen peas
- 2 tablespoons chopped fresh cilantro
- salt and freshly ground black pepper
- 2 tablespoons butter, melted
- mango chutney, for serving

Directions:

1. Start by making the dough. Combine the flour, baking powder, salt, pepper and dried thyme in a mixing bowl or the bowl of a stand mixer. Drizzle in the canola oil and pinch it together with your fingers to turn the flour into a crumby mixture. Stir in the water (enough to bring the dough together). Knead the dough for 5 minutes or so until it is smooth. Add a little more water or flour as needed. Let the dough rest while you make the turnover filling.

2. Preheat a large skillet on the stovetop over medium-high heat. Add the oil and sauté the onion until it starts to become tender – about 4 minutes. Add the garlic and ginger and continue to cook for another minute. Add the dried spices and toss everything to coat. Add the potatoes and cauliflower to the skillet and pour in 1½ cups of water. Simmer everything together for 20 to 25 minutes, or until the potatoes are soft and most of the water has evaporated. If the water has evaporated and the vegetables still need more time, just add a little water and continue to simmer until everything is tender. Stir well, crushing the potatoes and cauliflower a little as you do so. Stir in the peas and cilantro, season to taste with salt and freshly ground black pepper and set aside to cool.

3. Divide the dough into 4 balls. Roll the dough balls out into ¼-inch thick circles. Divide the cooled potato filling between the dough circles, placing a mound of the filling on one side of each piece of dough, leaving an empty border around the edge of the dough. Brush the edges of the dough with a little water and fold one edge of circle over the filling to meet the other edge of the circle, creating a half moon. Pinch the edges

together with your fingers and then press the edge with the tines of a fork to decorate and seal.

4. Preheat the air fryer to 380°F.

5. Spray or brush the air fryer basket with oil. Brush the turnovers with the melted butter and place 2 turnovers into the air fryer basket. Air-fry for 15 minutes. Flip the turnovers over and air-fry for another 5 minutes. Repeat with the remaining 2 turnovers.

6. These will be very hot when they come out of the air fryer. Let them cool for at least 20 minutes before serving warm with mango chutney.

Lentil Fritters

Servings: 9
Cooking Time: 12 Minutes

Ingredients:

- 1 cup cooked red lentils
- 1 cup riced cauliflower
- ½ medium zucchini, shredded (about 1 cup)
- ¼ cup finely chopped onion
- ¼ teaspoon salt
- ¼ teaspoon black pepper
- ½ teaspoon garlic powder
- ¼ teaspoon paprika
- 1 large egg
- ⅓ cup quinoa flour

Directions:

1. Preheat the air fryer to 370°F.

2. In a large bowl, mix the lentils, cauliflower, zucchini, onion, salt, pepper, garlic powder, and paprika. Mix in the egg and flour until a thick dough forms.

3. Using a large spoon, form the dough into 9 large fritters.

4. Liberally spray the air fryer basket with olive oil. Place the fritters into the basket, leaving space around each fritter so you can flip them.

5. Cook for 6 minutes, flip, and cook another 6 minutes.

6. Remove from the air fryer and repeat with the remaining fritters. Serve warm with desired sauce and sides.

Black Bean Empanadas

Servings: 12
Cooking Time: 35 Minutes

Ingredients:

- 1½ cups all-purpose flour
- 1 cup whole-wheat flour
- 1 teaspoon salt
- ½ cup cold unsalted butter
- 1 egg
- ½ cup milk
- One 14.5-ounce can black beans, drained and rinsed
- ¼ cup chopped cilantro
- 1 cup shredded purple cabbage
- 1 cup shredded Monterey jack cheese
- ¼ cup salsa

Directions:

1. In a food processor, place the all-purpose flour, whole-wheat flour, salt, and butter into processor and process for 2 minutes, scraping down the sides of the food processor every 30 seconds. Add in the egg and blend for 30 seconds. Using the pulse button, add in the milk 1 tablespoon at a time, or until dough is moist enough to handle and be rolled into a ball. Let the dough rest at room temperature for 30 minutes.

2. Meanwhile, in a large bowl, mix together the black beans, cilantro, cabbage, Monterey Jack cheese, and salsa.

3. On a floured surface, cut the dough in half; then form a ball and cut each ball into 6 equal

pieces, totaling 12 equal pieces. Work with one piece at a time, and cover the remaining dough with a towel.

4. Roll out a piece of dough into a 6-inch round, much like a tortilla, ¼ inch thick. Place 4 tablespoons of filling in the center of the round, and fold over to form a half-circle. Using a fork, crimp the edges together and pierce the top for air holes. Repeat with the remaining dough and filling.

5. Preheat the air fryer to 350°F.

6. Working in batches, place 3 to 4 empanadas in the air fryer basket and spray with cooking spray. Cook for 4 minutes, flip over the empanadas and spray with cooking spray, and cook another 4 minutes.

Thai Peanut Veggie Burgers

Servings: 6
Cooking Time: 14 Minutes
Ingredients:
- One 15.5-ounce can cannellini beans
- 1 teaspoon minced garlic
- ¼ cup chopped onion
- 1 Thai chili pepper, sliced
- 2 tablespoons natural peanut butter
- ½ teaspoon black pepper
- ½ teaspoon salt
- ⅓ cup all-purpose flour (optional)
- ½ cup cooked quinoa
- 1 large carrot, grated
- 1 cup shredded red cabbage
- ¼ cup peanut dressing
- ¼ cup chopped cilantro
- 6 Hawaiian rolls
- 6 butterleaf lettuce leaves

Directions:
1. Preheat the air fryer to 350°F.

2. To a blender or food processor fitted with a metal blade, add the beans, garlic, onion, chili pepper, peanut butter, pepper, and salt. Pulse for 5 to 10 seconds. Do not over process. The mixture should be coarse, not smooth.

3. Remove from the blender or food processor and spoon into a large bowl. Mix in the cooked quinoa and carrots. At this point, the mixture should begin to hold together to form small patties. If the dough appears to be too sticky (meaning you likely processed a little too long), add the flour to hold the patties together.

4. Using a large spoon, form 8 equal patties out of the batter.

5. Liberally spray a metal trivet with olive oil spray and set in the air fryer basket. Place the patties into the basket, leaving enough space to be able to turn them with a spatula.

6. Cook for 7 minutes, flip, and cook another 7 minutes.

7. Remove from the heat and repeat with additional patties.

8. To serve, place the red cabbage in a bowl and toss with peanut dressing and cilantro. Place the veggie burger on a bun, and top with a slice of lettuce and cabbage slaw.

Mexican Twice Air-fried Sweet Potatoes

Servings: 2
Cooking Time: 42 Minutes
Ingredients:
- 2 large sweet potatoes
- olive oil
- salt and freshly ground black pepper
- ⅓ cup diced red onion
- ⅓ cup diced red bell pepper

- ½ cup canned black beans, drained and rinsed
- ½ cup corn kernels, fresh or frozen
- ½ teaspoon chili powder
- 1½ cups grated pepper jack cheese, divided
- Jalapeño peppers, sliced

Directions:

1. Preheat the air fryer to 400°F.

2. Rub the outside of the sweet potatoes with olive oil and season with salt and freshly ground black pepper. Transfer the potatoes into the air fryer basket and air-fry at 400°F for 30 minutes, rotating the potatoes a few times during the cooking process.

3. While the potatoes are air-frying, start the potato filling. Preheat a large sauté pan over medium heat on the stovetop. Add the onion and pepper and sauté for a few minutes, until the vegetables start to soften. Add the black beans, corn, and chili powder and sauté for another 3 minutes. Set the mixture aside.

4. Remove the sweet potatoes from the air fryer and let them rest for 5 minutes. Slice off one inch of the flattest side of both potatoes. Scrape the potato flesh out of the potatoes, leaving half an inch of potato flesh around the edge of the potato. Place all the potato flesh into a large bowl and mash it with a fork. Add the black bean mixture and 1 cup of the pepper jack cheese to the mashed sweet potatoes. Season with salt and freshly ground black pepper and mix well. Stuff the hollowed out potato shells with the black bean and sweet potato mixture, mounding the filling high in the potatoes.

5. Transfer the stuffed potatoes back into the air fryer basket and air-fry at 370°F for 10 minutes. Sprinkle the remaining cheese on top of each stuffed potato, lower the heat to 340°F and air-fry for an additional 2 minutes to melt the cheese.

Top with a couple slices of Jalapeño pepper and serve warm with a green salad.

Roasted Vegetable Stromboli

Servings: 2

Cooking Time: 29 Minutes

Ingredients:

- ½ onion, thinly sliced
- ½ red pepper, julienned
- ½ yellow pepper, julienned
- olive oil
- 1 small zucchini, thinly sliced
- 1 cup thinly sliced mushrooms
- 1½ cups chopped broccoli
- 1 teaspoon Italian seasoning
- salt and freshly ground black pepper
- ½ recipe of Blue Jean Chef Pizza dough (page 231) OR 1 (14-ounce) tube refrigerated pizza dough
- 2 cups grated mozzarella cheese
- ¼ cup grated Parmesan cheese
- ½ cup sliced black olives, optional
- dried oregano
- pizza or marinara sauce

Directions:

1. Preheat the air fryer to 400°F.

2. Toss the onions and peppers with a little olive oil and air-fry the vegetables for 7 minutes, shaking the basket once or twice while the vegetables cook. Add the zucchini, mushrooms, broccoli and Italian seasoning to the basket. Add a little more olive oil and season with salt and freshly ground black pepper. Air-fry for an additional 7 minutes, shaking the basket halfway through. Let the vegetables cool slightly while you roll out the pizza dough.

3. On a lightly floured surface, roll or press the pizza dough out into a 13-inch by 11-inch

rectangle, with the long side closest to you. Sprinkle half of the mozzarella and Parmesan cheeses over the dough leaving an empty 1-inch border from the edge farthest away from you. Spoon the roasted vegetables over the cheese, sprinkle the olives over everything and top with the remaining cheese.

4.   Start rolling the stromboli away from you and toward the empty border. Make sure the filling stays tightly tucked inside the roll. Finally, tuck the ends of the dough in and pinch the seam shut. Place the seam side down and shape the stromboli into a U-shape to fit into the air fryer basket. Cut 4 small slits with the tip of a sharp knife evenly in the top of the dough, lightly brush the stromboli with a little oil and sprinkle with some dried oregano.

5.   Preheat the air fryer to 360°F.

6.   Spray or brush the air fryer basket with oil and transfer the U-shaped stromboli to the air fryer basket. Air-fry for 15 minutes, flipping the stromboli over after the first 10 minutes. (Use a plate to invert the Stromboli out of the air fryer basket and then slide it back into the basket off the plate.)

7.   To remove, carefully flip the stromboli over onto a cutting board. Let it rest for a couple of minutes before serving. Cut it into 2-inch slices and serve with pizza or marinara sauce.

Roasted Vegetable Thai Green Curry

Servings: 4

Cooking Time: 16 Minutes

Ingredients:

- 1 (13-ounce) can coconut milk
- 3 tablespoons green curry paste
- 1 tablespoon soy sauce*
- 1 tablespoon rice wine vinegar
- 1 teaspoon sugar
- 1 teaspoon minced fresh ginger
- ½ onion, chopped
- 3 carrots, sliced
- 1 red bell pepper, chopped
- olive oil
- 10 stalks of asparagus, cut into 2-inch pieces
- 3 cups broccoli florets
- basmati rice for serving
- fresh cilantro
- crushed red pepper flakes (optional)

Directions:

1.   Combine the coconut milk, green curry paste, soy sauce, rice wine vinegar, sugar and ginger in a medium saucepan and bring to a boil on the stovetop. Reduce the heat and simmer for 20 minutes while you cook the vegetables. Set aside.

2.   Preheat the air fryer to 400°F.

3.   Toss the onion, carrots, and red pepper together with a little olive oil and transfer the vegetables to the air fryer basket. Air-fry at 400°F for 10 minutes, shaking the basket a few times during the cooking process. Add the asparagus and broccoli florets and air-fry for an additional 6 minutes, again shaking the basket for even cooking.

4.   When the vegetables are cooked to your liking, toss them with the green curry sauce and serve in bowls over basmati rice. Garnish with fresh chopped cilantro and crushed red pepper flakes.

Roasted Vegetable Lasagna

Servings: 6
Cooking Time: 55 Minutes

Ingredients:

- 1 zucchini, sliced
- 1 yellow squash, sliced
- 8 ounces mushrooms, sliced
- 1 red bell pepper, cut into 2-inch strips
- 1 tablespoon olive oil
- 2 cups ricotta cheese
- 2 cups grated mozzarella cheese, divided
- 1 egg
- 1 teaspoon salt
- freshly ground black pepper
- ¼ cup shredded carrots
- ½ cup chopped fresh spinach
- 8 lasagna noodles, cooked
- Béchamel Sauce:
- 3 tablespoons butter
- 3 tablespoons flour
- 2½ cups milk
- ½ cup grated Parmesan cheese
- ½ teaspoon salt
- freshly ground black pepper
- pinch of ground nutmeg

Directions:

1. Preheat the air fryer to 400°F.

2. Toss the zucchini, yellow squash, mushrooms and red pepper in a large bowl with the olive oil and season with salt and pepper. Air-fry for 10 minutes, shaking the basket once or twice while the vegetables cook.

3. While the vegetables are cooking, make the béchamel sauce and cheese filling. Melt the butter in a medium saucepan over medium-high heat on the stovetop. Add the flour and whisk, cooking for a couple of minutes. Add the milk and whisk vigorously until smooth. Bring the mixture to a boil and simmer until the sauce thickens. Stir in the Parmesan cheese and season with the salt, pepper and nutmeg. Set the sauce aside.

4. Combine the ricotta cheese, 1¼ cups of the mozzarella cheese, egg, salt and pepper in a large bowl and stir until combined. Fold in the carrots and spinach.

5. When the vegetables have finished cooking, build the lasagna. Use a baking dish that is 6 inches in diameter and 4 inches high. Cover the bottom of the baking dish with a little béchamel sauce. Top with two lasagna noodles, cut to fit the dish and overlapping each other a little. Spoon a third of the ricotta cheese mixture and then a third of the roasted veggies on top of the noodles. Pour ½ cup of béchamel sauce on top and then repeat these layers two more times: noodles – cheese mixture – vegetables – béchamel sauce. Sprinkle the remaining mozzarella cheese over the top. Cover the dish with aluminum foil, tenting it loosely so the aluminum doesn't touch the cheese.

6. Lower the dish into the air fryer basket using an aluminum foil sling (fold a piece of aluminum foil into a strip about 2-inches wide by 24-inches long). Fold the ends of the aluminum foil over the top of the dish before returning the basket to the air fryer. Air-fry for 45 minutes, removing the foil for the last 2 minutes, to slightly brown the cheese on top.

7. Let the lasagna rest for at least 20 minutes to set up a little before slicing into it and serving.

Arancini With Marinara

Servings: 6

Cooking Time: 15 Minutes

Ingredients:

- 2 cups cooked rice
- 1 cup grated Parmesan cheese
- 1 egg, whisked
- ¼ teaspoon dried thyme
- ½ teaspoon dried oregano
- ½ teaspoon dried basil
- ½ teaspoon dried parsley
- 1 teaspoon salt
- ¼ teaspoon paprika
- 1 cup breadcrumbs
- 4 ounces mozzarella, cut into 24 cubes
- 2 cups marinara sauce

Directions:

1. In a large bowl, mix together the rice, Parmesan cheese, and egg.

2. In another bowl, mix together the thyme, oregano, basil, parsley, salt, paprika, and breadcrumbs.

3. Form 24 rice balls with the rice mixture. Use your thumb to make an indentation in the center and stuff 1 cube of mozzarella in the center of the rice; close the ball around the cheese.

4. Roll the rice balls in the seasoned breadcrumbs until all are coated.

5. Preheat the air fryer to 400°F.

6. Place the rice balls in the air fryer basket and coat with cooking spray. Cook for 8 minutes, shake the basket, and cook another 7 minutes.

7. Heat the marinara sauce in a saucepan until warm. Serve sauce as a dip for arancini.

Falafel

Servings: 4

Cooking Time: 10 Minutes

Ingredients:

- 1 cup dried chickpeas
- ½ onion, chopped
- 1 clove garlic
- ¼ cup fresh parsley leaves
- 1 teaspoon salt
- ¼ teaspoon crushed red pepper flakes
- 1 teaspoon ground cumin
- ½ teaspoon ground coriander
- 1 to 2 tablespoons flour
- olive oil
- Tomato Salad
- 2 tomatoes, seeds removed and diced
- ½ cucumber, finely diced
- ¼ red onion, finely diced and rinsed with water
- 1 teaspoon red wine vinegar
- 1 tablespoon olive oil
- salt and freshly ground black pepper
- 2 tablespoons chopped fresh parsley

Directions:

1. Cover the chickpeas with water and let them soak overnight on the counter. Then drain the chickpeas and put them in a food processor, along with the onion, garlic, parsley, spices and 1 tablespoon of flour. Pulse in the food processor until the mixture has broken down into a coarse paste consistency. The mixture should hold together when you pinch it. Add more flour as needed, until you get this consistency.

2. Scoop portions of the mixture (about 2 tablespoons in size) and shape into balls. Place the balls on a plate and refrigerate for at least 30 minutes. You should have between 12 and 14 balls.

3. Preheat the air fryer to 380°F.

4. Spray the falafel balls with oil and place them in the air fryer. Air-fry for 10 minutes, rolling them over and spraying them with oil again halfway through the cooking time so that they cook and brown evenly.

5. Serve with pita bread, hummus, cucumbers, hot peppers, tomatoes or any other fillings you might like.

Rigatoni With Roasted Onions, Fennel, Spinach And Lemon Pepper Ricotta

Servings: 2
Cooking Time: 13 Minutes
Ingredients:
- 1 red onion, rough chopped into large chunks
- 2 teaspoons olive oil, divided
- 1 bulb fennel, sliced ¼-inch thick
- ¾ cup ricotta cheese
- 1½ teaspoons finely chopped lemon zest, plus more for garnish
- 1 teaspoon lemon juice
- salt and freshly ground black pepper
- 8 ounces (½ pound) dried rigatoni pasta
- 3 cups baby spinach leaves

Directions:
1. Bring a large stockpot of salted water to a boil on the stovetop and Preheat the air fryer to 400°F.
2. While the water is coming to a boil, toss the chopped onion in 1 teaspoon of olive oil and transfer to the air fryer basket. Air-fry at 400°F for 5 minutes. Toss the sliced fennel with 1 teaspoon of olive oil and add this to the air fryer basket with the onions. Continue to air-fry at 400°F for 8 minutes, shaking the basket a few times during the cooking process.

3. Combine the ricotta cheese, lemon zest and juice, ¼ teaspoon of salt and freshly ground black pepper in a bowl and stir until smooth.
4. Add the dried rigatoni to the boiling water and cook according to the package directions. When the pasta is cooked al dente, reserve one cup of the pasta water and drain the pasta into a colander.
5. Place the spinach in a serving bowl and immediately transfer the hot pasta to the bowl, wilting the spinach. Add the roasted onions and fennel and toss together. Add a little pasta water to the dish if it needs moistening. Then, dollop the lemon pepper ricotta cheese on top and nestle it into the hot pasta. Garnish with more lemon zest if desired.

Roasted Vegetable Pita Pizza

Servings: 4
Cooking Time: 20 Minutes
Ingredients:
- 1 medium red bell pepper, seeded and cut into quarters
- 1 teaspoon extra-virgin olive oil
- ⅛ teaspoon black pepper
- ⅛ teaspoon salt
- Two 6-inch whole-grain pita breads
- 6 tablespoons pesto sauce
- ¼ small red onion, thinly sliced
- ½ cup shredded part-skim mozzarella cheese

Directions:
1. Preheat the air fryer to 400°F.
2. In a small bowl, toss the bell peppers with the olive oil, pepper, and salt.
3. Place the bell peppers in the air fryer and cook for 15 minutes, shaking every 5 minutes to prevent burning.

4. Remove the peppers and set aside. Turn the air fryer temperature down to 350°F.

5. Lay the pita bread on a flat surface. Cover each with half the pesto sauce; then top with even portions of the red bell peppers and onions. Sprinkle cheese over the top. Spray the air fryer basket with olive oil mist.

6. Carefully lift the pita bread into the air fryer basket with a spatula.

7. Cook for 5 to 8 minutes, or until the outer edges begin to brown and the cheese is melted.

8. Serve warm with desired sides.

Charred Cauliflower Tacos

Servings: 4

Cooking Time: 10 Minutes

Ingredients:

- 1 head cauliflower, washed and cut into florets
- 2 tablespoons avocado oil
- 2 teaspoons taco seasoning
- 1 medium avocado
- ½ teaspoon garlic powder
- ¼ teaspoon black pepper
- ¼ teaspoon salt
- 2 tablespoons chopped red onion
- 2 teaspoons fresh squeezed lime juice
- ¼ cup chopped cilantro
- Eight 6-inch corn tortillas
- ½ cup cooked corn
- ½ cup shredded purple cabbage

Directions:

1. Preheat the air fryer to 390°F.

2. In a large bowl, toss the cauliflower with the avocado oil and taco seasoning. Set the metal trivet inside the air fryer basket and liberally spray with olive oil.

3. Place the cauliflower onto the trivet and cook for 10 minutes, shaking every 3 minutes to allow for an even char.

4. While the cauliflower is cooking, prepare the avocado sauce. In a medium bowl, mash the avocado; then mix in the garlic powder, pepper, salt, and onion. Stir in the lime juice and cilantro; set aside.

5. Remove the cauliflower from the air fryer basket.

6. Place 1 tablespoon of avocado sauce in the middle of a tortilla, and top with corn, cabbage, and charred cauliflower. Repeat with the remaining tortillas. Serve immediately.

Veggie Burgers

Servings: 4

Cooking Time: 15 Minutes

Ingredients:

- 2 cans black beans, rinsed and drained
- ½ cup cooked quinoa
- ½ cup shredded raw sweet potato
- ¼ cup diced red onion
- 2 teaspoons ground cumin
- 1 teaspoon coriander powder
- ½ teaspoon salt
- oil for misting or cooking spray
- 8 slices bread
- suggested toppings: lettuce, tomato, red onion, Pepper Jack cheese, guacamole

Directions:

1. In a medium bowl, mash the beans with a fork.

2. Add the quinoa, sweet potato, onion, cumin, coriander, and salt and mix well with the fork.

3. Shape into 4 patties, each ¾-inch thick.

4. Mist both sides with oil or cooking spray and also mist the basket.

5. Cook at 390°F for 15minutes.

6. Follow the recipe for Toast, Plain & Simple.

7. Pop the veggie burgers back in the air fryer for a minute or two to reheat if necessary.

8. Serve on the toast with your favorite burger toppings.

Tacos

Servings: 24

Cooking Time: 8 Minutes Per Batch

Ingredients:

- 1 24-count package 4-inch corn tortillas
- 1½ cups refried beans (about ¾ of a 15-ounce can)
- 4 ounces sharp Cheddar cheese, grated
- ½ cup salsa
- oil for misting or cooking spray

Directions:

1. Preheat air fryer to 390°F.

2. Wrap refrigerated tortillas in damp paper towels and microwave for 30 to 60 seconds to warm. If necessary, rewarm tortillas as you go to keep them soft enough to fold without breaking.

3. Working with one tortilla at a time, top with 1 tablespoon of beans, 1 tablespoon of grated cheese, and 1 teaspoon of salsa. Fold over and press down very gently on the center. Press edges firmly all around to seal. Spray both sides with oil or cooking spray.

4. Cooking in two batches, place half the tacos in the air fryer basket. To cook 12 at a time, you may need to stand them upright and lean some against the sides of basket. It's okay if they're crowded as long as you leave a little room for air to circulate around them.

5. Cook for 8 minutes or until golden brown and crispy.

6. Repeat steps 4 and 5 to cook remaining tacos.

Cheese Ravioli

Servings: 4

Cooking Time: 9 Minutes

Ingredients:

- 1 egg
- ¼ cup milk
- 1 cup breadcrumbs
- 2 teaspoons Italian seasoning
- ⅛ teaspoon ground rosemary
- ¼ teaspoon basil
- ¼ teaspoon parsley
- 9-ounce package uncooked cheese ravioli
- ¼ cup flour
- oil for misting or cooking spray

Directions:

1. Preheat air fryer to 390°F.

2. In a medium bowl, beat together egg and milk.

3. In a large plastic bag, mix together the breadcrumbs, Italian seasoning, rosemary, basil, and parsley.

4. Place all the ravioli and the flour in a bag or a bowl with a lid and shake to coat.

5. Working with a handful at a time, drop floured ravioli into egg wash. Remove ravioli, letting excess drip off, and place in bag with breadcrumbs.

6. When all ravioli are in the breadcrumbs' bag, shake well to coat all pieces.

7. Dump enough ravioli into air fryer basket to form one layer. Mist with oil or cooking spray. Dump the remaining ravioli on top of the first layer and mist with oil.

8. Cook for 5minutes. Shake well and spray with oil. Break apart any ravioli stuck together and spray any spots you missed the first time.

9. Cook 4 minutes longer, until ravioli puff up and are crispy golden brown.

Corn And Pepper Jack Chile Rellenos With Roasted Tomato Sauce

Servings: 3

Cooking Time: 30 Minutes

Ingredients:

- 3 Poblano peppers
- 1 cup all-purpose flour*
- salt and freshly ground black pepper
- 2 eggs, lightly beaten
- 1 cup plain breadcrumbs*
- olive oil, in a spray bottle
- Sauce
- 2 cups cherry tomatoes
- 1 Jalapeño pepper, halved and seeded
- 1 clove garlic
- ¼ red onion, broken into large pieces
- 1 tablespoon olive oil
- salt, to taste
- 2 tablespoons chopped fresh cilantro
- Filling
- olive oil
- ¼ red onion, finely chopped
- 1 teaspoon minced garlic
- 1 cup corn kernels, fresh or frozen
- 2 cups grated pepper jack cheese

Directions:

1. Start by roasting the peppers. Preheat the air fryer to 400°F. Place the peppers into the air fryer basket and air-fry at 400°F for 10 minutes, turning them over halfway through the cooking time. Remove the peppers from the basket and cover loosely with foil.

2. While the peppers are cooling, make the roasted tomato sauce. Place all sauce Ingredients except for the cilantro into the air fryer basket and air-fry at 400°F for 10 minutes, shaking the basket once or twice. When the sauce Ingredients have finished air-frying, transfer everything to a blender or food processor and blend or process to a smooth sauce, adding a little warm water to get the desired consistency. Season to taste with salt, add the cilantro and set aside.

3. While the sauce Ingredients are cooking in the air fryer, make the filling. Heat a skillet on the stovetop over medium heat. Add the olive oil and sauté the red onion and garlic for 4 to 5 minutes. Transfer the onion and garlic to a bowl, stir in the corn and cheese, and set aside.

4. Set up a dredging station with three shallow dishes. Place the flour, seasoned with salt and pepper, in the first shallow dish. Place the eggs in the second dish, and fill the third shallow dish with the breadcrumbs. When the peppers have cooled, carefully slice into one side of the pepper to create an opening. Pull the seeds out of the peppers and peel away the skins, trying not to tear the pepper. Fill each pepper with some of the corn and cheese filling and close the pepper up again by folding one side of the opening over the other. Carefully roll each pepper in the seasoned flour, then into the egg and finally into the breadcrumbs to coat on all sides, trying not to let the pepper fall open. Spray the peppers on all sides with a little olive oil.

5. Air-fry two peppers at a time at 350°F for 6 minutes. Turn the peppers over and air-fry for another 4 minutes. Serve the peppers warm on a bed of the roasted tomato sauce.

Eggplant Parmesan

Servings: 4

Cooking Time: 8 Minutes Per Batch

Ingredients:

- 1 medium eggplant, 6–8 inches long
- salt
- 1 large egg
- 1 tablespoon water
- ⅔ cup panko breadcrumbs
- ⅓ cup grated Parmesan cheese, plus more for serving
- 1 tablespoon Italian seasoning
- ¾ teaspoon oregano
- oil for misting or cooking spray
- 1 24-ounce jar marinara sauce
- 8 ounces spaghetti, cooked
- pepper

Directions:

1. Preheat air fryer to 390°F.

2. Leaving peel intact, cut eggplant into 8 round slices about ¾-inch thick. Salt to taste.

3. Beat egg and water in a shallow dish.

4. In another shallow dish, combine panko, Parmesan, Italian seasoning, and oregano.

5. Dip eggplant slices in egg wash and then crumbs, pressing lightly to coat.

6. Mist slices with oil or cooking spray.

7. Place 4 eggplant slices in air fryer basket and cook for 8 minutes, until brown and crispy.

8. While eggplant is cooking, heat marinara sauce.

9. Repeat step 7 to cook remaining eggplant slices.

10. To serve, place cooked spaghetti on plates and top with marinara and eggplant slices. At the table, pass extra Parmesan cheese and freshly ground black pepper.

Parmesan Portobello Mushroom Caps

Servings: 2

Cooking Time: 14 Minutes

Ingredients:

- ¼ cup flour*
- 1 egg, lightly beaten
- 1 cup seasoned breadcrumbs*
- 2 large portobello mushroom caps, stems and gills removed
- olive oil, in a spray bottle
- ½ cup tomato sauce
- ¾ cup grated mozzarella cheese
- 1 tablespoon grated Parmesan cheese
- 1 tablespoon chopped fresh basil or parsley

Directions:

1. Set up a dredging station with three shallow dishes. Place the flour in the first shallow dish, egg in the second dish and breadcrumbs in the last dish. Dredge the mushrooms in flour, then dip them into the egg and finally press them into the breadcrumbs to coat on all sides. Spray both sides of the coated mushrooms with olive oil.

2. Preheat the air fryer to 400°F.

3. Air-fry the mushrooms at 400°F for 10 minutes, turning them over halfway through the cooking process.

4. Fill the underside of the mushrooms with the tomato sauce and then top the sauce with the mozzarella and Parmesan cheeses. Reset the air fryer temperature to 350°F and air-fry for an additional 4 minutes, until the cheese has melted and is slightly browned.

5. Serve the mushrooms with pasta tossed with tomato sauce and garnish with some chopped fresh basil or parsley.

Vegetable Couscous

Servings: 4

Cooking Time: 10 Minutes

Ingredients:

- 4 ounces white mushrooms, sliced
- ½ medium green bell pepper, julienned
- 1 cup cubed zucchini
- ¼ small onion, slivered
- 1 stalk celery, thinly sliced
- ¼ teaspoon ground coriander
- ¼ teaspoon ground cumin
- salt and pepper
- 1 tablespoon olive oil
- Couscous
- ¾ cup uncooked couscous
- 1 cup vegetable broth or water
- ½ teaspoon salt (omit if using salted broth)

Directions:

1. Combine all vegetables in large bowl. Sprinkle with coriander, cumin, and salt and pepper to taste. Stir well, add olive oil, and stir again to coat vegetables evenly.

2. Place vegetables in air fryer basket and cook at 390°F for 5minutes. Stir and cook for 5 more minutes, until tender.

3. While vegetables are cooking, prepare the couscous: Place broth or water and salt in large saucepan. Heat to boiling, stir in couscous, cover, and remove from heat.

4. Let couscous sit for 5minutes, stir in cooked vegetables, and serve hot.

Spicy Sesame Tempeh Slaw With Peanut Dressing

Servings: 2

Cooking Time: 8 Minutes

Ingredients:

- 2 cups hot water
- 1 teaspoon salt
- 8 ounces tempeh, sliced into 1-inch-long pieces
- 2 tablespoons low-sodium soy sauce
- 2 tablespoons rice vinegar
- 1 tablespoon filtered water
- 2 teaspoons sesame oil
- ½ teaspoon fresh ginger
- 1 clove garlic, minced
- ¼ teaspoon black pepper
- ½ jalapeño, sliced
- 4 cups cabbage slaw
- 4 tablespoons Peanut Dressing (see the following recipe)
- 2 tablespoons fresh chopped cilantro
- 2 tablespoons chopped peanuts

Directions:

1. Mix the hot water with the salt and pour over the tempeh in a glass bowl. Stir and cover with a towel for 10 minutes.

2. Discard the water and leave the tempeh in the bowl.

3. In a medium bowl, mix the soy sauce, rice vinegar, filtered water, sesame oil, ginger, garlic, pepper, and jalapeño. Pour over the tempeh and cover with a towel. Place in the refrigerator to marinate for at least 2 hours.

4. Preheat the air fryer to 370°F. Remove the tempeh from the bowl and discard the remaining marinade.

5. Liberally spray the metal trivet that goes into the air fryer basket and place the tempeh on top of the trivet.

6. Cook for 4 minutes, flip, and cook another 4 minutes.

7. In a large bowl, mix the cabbage slaw with the Peanut Dressing and toss in the cilantro and chopped peanuts.

8. Portion onto 4 plates and place the cooked tempeh on top when cooking completes. Serve immediately.

Mushroom, Zucchini And Black Bean Burgers

Servings: 4

Cooking Time: 18 Minutes

Ingredients:

- 1 cup diced zucchini, (about ½ medium zucchini)
- 1 tablespoon olive oil
- salt and freshly ground black pepper
- 1 cup chopped brown mushrooms (about 3 ounces)
- 1 small clove garlic
- 1 (15-ounce) can black beans, drained and rinsed
- 1 teaspoon lemon zest
- 1 tablespoon chopped fresh cilantro
- ½ cup plain breadcrumbs
- 1 egg, beaten
- ½ teaspoon salt
- freshly ground black pepper
- whole-wheat pita bread, burger buns or brioche buns
- mayonnaise, tomato, avocado and lettuce, for serving

Directions:

1. Preheat the air fryer to 400°F.

2. Toss the zucchini with the olive oil, season with salt and freshly ground black pepper and air-fry for 6 minutes, shaking the basket once or twice while it cooks.

3. Transfer the zucchini to a food processor with the mushrooms, garlic and black beans and process until still a little chunky but broken down and pasty. Transfer the mixture to a bowl. Add the lemon zest, cilantro, breadcrumbs and egg and mix well. Season again with salt and freshly ground black pepper. Shape the mixture into four burger patties and refrigerate for at least 15 minutes.

4. Preheat the air fryer to 370°F. Transfer two of the veggie burgers to the air fryer basket and air-fry for 12 minutes, flipping the burgers gently halfway through the cooking time. Keep the burgers warm by loosely tenting them with foil while you cook the remaining two burgers. Return the first batch of burgers back into the air fryer with the second batch for the last two minutes of cooking to re-heat.

5. Serve on toasted whole-wheat pita bread, burger buns or brioche buns with some mayonnaise, tomato, avocado and lettuce.

Cauliflower Steaks Gratin

Servings: 2

Cooking Time: 13 Minutes

Ingredients:

- 1 head cauliflower
- 1 tablespoon olive oil
- salt and freshly ground black pepper
- ½ teaspoon chopped fresh thyme leaves
- 3 tablespoons grated Parmigiano-Reggiano cheese
- 2 tablespoons panko breadcrumbs

Directions:

1. Preheat the air-fryer to 370°F.

2. Cut two steaks out of the center of the cauliflower. To do this, cut the cauliflower in half and then cut one slice about 1-inch thick off each

half. The rest of the cauliflower will fall apart into florets, which you can roast on their own or save for another meal.

3. Brush both sides of the cauliflower steaks with olive oil and season with salt, freshly ground black pepper and fresh thyme. Place the cauliflower steaks into the air fryer basket and air-fry for 6 minutes. Turn the steaks over and air-fry for another 4 minutes. Combine the Parmesan cheese and panko breadcrumbs and sprinkle the mixture over the tops of both steaks and air-fry for another 3 minutes until the cheese has melted and the breadcrumbs have browned. Serve this with some sautéed bitter greens and air-fried blistered tomatoes.

Spinach And Cheese Calzone

Servings: 2
Cooking Time: 10 Minutes
Ingredients:
- ⅔ cup frozen chopped spinach, thawed
- 1 cup grated mozzarella cheese
- 1 cup ricotta cheese
- ½ teaspoon Italian seasoning
- ½ teaspoon salt
- freshly ground black pepper
- 1 store-bought or homemade pizza dough* (about 12 to 16 ounces)
- 2 tablespoons olive oil
- pizza or marinara sauce (optional)

Directions:
1. Drain and squeeze all the water out of the thawed spinach and set it aside. Mix the mozzarella cheese, ricotta cheese, Italian seasoning, salt and freshly ground black pepper together in a bowl. Stir in the chopped spinach.
2. Divide the dough in half. With floured hands or on a floured surface, stretch or roll one half of the dough into a 10-inch circle. Spread half of the cheese and spinach mixture on half of the dough, leaving about one inch of dough empty around the edge.

3. Fold the other half of the dough over the cheese mixture, almost to the edge of the bottom dough to form a half moon. Fold the bottom edge of dough up over the top edge and crimp the dough around the edges in order to make the crust and seal the calzone. Brush the dough with olive oil. Repeat with the second half of dough to make the second calzone.

4. Preheat the air fryer to 360°F.

5. Brush or spray the air fryer basket with olive oil. Air-fry the calzones one at a time for 10 minutes, flipping the calzone over half way through. Serve with warm pizza or marinara sauce if desired.

Asparagus, Mushroom And Cheese Soufflés

Servings: 3
Cooking Time: 21 Minutes
Ingredients:
- butter
- grated Parmesan cheese
- 3 button mushrooms, thinly sliced
- 8 spears asparagus, sliced ½-inch long
- 1 teaspoon olive oil
- 1 tablespoon butter
- 4½ teaspoons flour
- pinch paprika
- pinch ground nutmeg
- salt and freshly ground black pepper
- ½ cup milk
- ½ cup grated Gruyère cheese or other Swiss cheese (about 2 ounces)

- 2 eggs, separated

Directions:

1. Butter three 6-ounce ramekins and dust with grated Parmesan cheese. (Butter the ramekins and then coat the butter with Parmesan by shaking it around in the ramekin and dumping out any excess.)

2. Preheat the air fryer to 400°F.

3. Toss the mushrooms and asparagus in a bowl with the olive oil. Transfer the vegetables to the air fryer and air-fry for 7 minutes, shaking the basket once or twice to redistribute the Ingredients while they cook.

4. While the vegetables are cooking, make the soufflé base. Melt the butter in a saucepan on the stovetop over medium heat. Add the flour, stir and cook for a minute or two. Add the paprika, nutmeg, salt and pepper. Whisk in the milk and bring the mixture to a simmer to thicken. Remove the pan from the heat and add the cheese, stirring to melt. Let the mixture cool for just a few minutes and then whisk the egg yolks in, one at a time. Stir in the cooked mushrooms and asparagus. Let this soufflé base cool.

5. In a separate bowl, whisk the egg whites to soft peak stage (the point at which the whites can almost stand up on the end of your whisk). Fold the whipped egg whites into the soufflé base, adding a little at a time.

6. Preheat the air fryer to 330°F.

7. Transfer the batter carefully to the buttered ramekins, leaving about ½-inch at the top. Place the ramekins into the air fryer basket and air-fry for 14 minutes. The soufflés should have risen nicely and be brown on top. Serve immediately.

Roasted Vegetable, Brown Rice And Black Bean Burrito

Servings: 2

Cooking Time: 20 Minutes

Ingredients:

- ½ zucchini, sliced ¼-inch thick
- ½ red onion, sliced
- 1 yellow bell pepper, sliced
- 2 teaspoons olive oil
- salt and freshly ground black pepper
- 2 burrito size flour tortillas
- 1 cup grated pepper jack cheese
- ½ cup cooked brown rice
- ½ cup canned black beans, drained and rinsed
- ¼ teaspoon ground cumin
- 1 tablespoon chopped fresh cilantro
- fresh salsa, guacamole and sour cream, for serving

Directions:

1. Preheat the air fryer to 400°F.

2. Toss the vegetables in a bowl with the olive oil, salt and freshly ground black pepper. Air-fry at 400°F for 12 to 15 minutes, shaking the basket a few times during the cooking process. The vegetables are done when they are cooked to your liking.

3. In the meantime, start building the burritos. Lay the tortillas out on the counter. Sprinkle half of the cheese in the center of the tortillas. Combine the rice, beans, cumin and cilantro in a bowl, season to taste with salt and freshly ground black pepper and then divide the mixture between the two tortillas. When the vegetables have finished cooking, transfer them to the two tortillas, placing the vegetables on top of the rice and beans. Sprinkle the remaining cheese on top and then roll the burritos up, tucking in the sides

of the tortillas as you roll. Brush or spray the outside of the burritos with olive oil and transfer them to the air fryer.

4. Air-fry at 360°F for 8 minutes, turning them over when there are about 2 minutes left. The burritos will have slightly brown spots, but will still be pliable.

5. Serve with some fresh salsa, guacamole and sour cream.

Basic Fried Tofu

Servings: 4

Cooking Time: 17 Minutes

Ingredients:

- 14 ounces extra-firm tofu, drained and pressed
- 1 tablespoon sesame oil
- 2 tablespoons low-sodium soy sauce
- ¼ cup rice vinegar
- 1 tablespoon fresh grated ginger
- 1 clove garlic, minced
- 3 tablespoons cornstarch
- ¼ teaspoon black pepper
- ⅛ teaspoon salt

Directions:

1. Cut the tofu into 16 cubes. Set aside in a glass container with a lid.

2. In a medium bowl, mix the sesame oil, soy sauce, rice vinegar, ginger, and garlic. Pour over the tofu and secure the lid. Place in the refrigerator to marinate for an hour.

3. Preheat the air fryer to 350°F.

4. In a small bowl, mix the cornstarch, black pepper, and salt.

5. Transfer the tofu to a large bowl and discard the leftover marinade. Pour the cornstarch mixture over the tofu and toss until all the pieces are coated.

6. Liberally spray the air fryer basket with olive oil mist and set the tofu pieces inside. Allow space between the tofu so it can cook evenly. Cook in batches if necessary.

7. Cook 15 to 17 minutes, shaking the basket every 5 minutes to allow the tofu to cook evenly on all sides. When it's done cooking, the tofu will be crisped and browned on all sides.

8. Remove the tofu from the air fryer basket and serve warm.

Tandoori Paneer Naan Pizza

Servings: 4

Cooking Time: 10 Minutes

Ingredients:

- 6 tablespoons plain Greek yogurt, divided
- 1¼ teaspoons garam marsala, divided
- ½ teaspoon turmeric, divided
- ¼ teaspoon garlic powder
- ½ teaspoon paprika, divided
- ½ teaspoon black pepper, divided
- 3 ounces paneer, cut into small cubes
- 1 tablespoon extra-virgin olive oil
- 2 teaspoons minced garlic
- 4 cups baby spinach
- 2 tablespoons marinara sauce
- ¼ teaspoon salt
- 2 plain naan breads (approximately 6 inches in diameter)
- ½ cup shredded part-skim mozzarella cheese

Directions:

1. Preheat the air fryer to 350°F.

2. In a small bowl, mix 2 tablespoons of the yogurt, ½ teaspoon of the garam marsala, ¼ teaspoon of the turmeric, the garlic powder, ¼ teaspoon of the paprika, and ¼ teaspoon of the black pepper. Toss the paneer cubes in the mixture and let marinate for at least an hour.

3. Meanwhile, in a pan, heat the olive oil over medium heat. Add in the minced garlic and sauté for 1 minute. Stir in the spinach and begin to cook until it wilts. Add in the remaining 4 tablespoons of yogurt and the marinara sauce. Stir in the remaining ¾ teaspoon of garam masala, the remaining ¼ teaspoon of turmeric, the remaining ¼ teaspoon of paprika, the remaining ¼ teaspoon of black pepper, and the salt. Let simmer a minute or two, and then remove from the heat.

4. Equally divide the spinach mixture amongst the two naan breads. Place 1½ ounces of the marinated paneer on each naan.

5. Liberally spray the air fryer basket with olive oil mist.

6. Use a spatula to pick up one naan and place it in the air fryer basket.

7. Cook for 4 minutes, open the basket and sprinkle ¼ cup of mozzarella cheese on top, and cook another 4 minutes.

8. Remove from the air fryer and repeat with the remaining naan.

9. Serve warm.

Spicy Vegetable And Tofu Shake Fry

Servings: 4
Cooking Time: 17 Minutes
Ingredients:
- 4 teaspoons canola oil, divided
- 2 tablespoons rice wine vinegar
- 1 tablespoon sriracha chili sauce
- ¼ cup soy sauce*
- ½ teaspoon toasted sesame oil
- 1 teaspoon minced garlic
- 1 tablespoon minced fresh ginger
- 8 ounces extra firm tofu
- ½ cup vegetable stock or water
- 1 tablespoon honey
- 1 tablespoon cornstarch
- ½ red onion, chopped
- 1 red or yellow bell pepper, chopped
- 1 cup green beans, cut into 2-inch lengths
- 4 ounces mushrooms, sliced
- 2 scallions, sliced
- 2 tablespoons fresh cilantro leaves
- 2 teaspoons toasted sesame seeds

Directions:
1. Combine 1 tablespoon of the oil, vinegar, sriracha sauce, soy sauce, sesame oil, garlic and ginger in a small bowl. Cut the tofu into bite-sized cubes and toss the tofu in with the marinade while you prepare the other vegetables. When you are ready to start cooking, remove the tofu from the marinade and set it aside. Add the water, honey and cornstarch to the marinade and bring to a simmer on the stovetop, just until the sauce thickens. Set the sauce aside.

2. Preheat the air fryer to 400°F.

3. Toss the onion, pepper, green beans and mushrooms in a bowl with a little canola oil and season with salt. Air-fry at 400°F for 11 minutes, shaking the basket and tossing the vegetables every few minutes. When the vegetables are cooked to your preferred doneness, remove them from the air fryer and set aside.

4. Add the tofu to the air fryer basket and air-fry at 400°F for 6 minutes, shaking the basket a few times during the cooking process. Add the vegetables back to the basket and air-fry for another minute. Transfer the vegetables and tofu to a large bowl, add the scallions and cilantro leaves and toss with the sauce. Serve over rice with sesame seeds sprinkled on top.

Sandwiches And Burgers Recipes

Best-ever Roast Beef Sandwiches

Servings: 6
Cooking Time: 30-50 Minutes
Ingredients:
- 2½ teaspoons Olive oil
- 1½ teaspoons Dried oregano
- 1½ teaspoons Dried thyme
- 1½ teaspoons Onion powder
- 1½ teaspoons Table salt
- 1½ teaspoons Ground black pepper
- 3 pounds Beef eye of round
- 6 Round soft rolls, such as Kaiser rolls or hamburger buns (gluten-free, if a concern), split open lengthwise
- ¾ cup Regular, low-fat, or fat-free mayonnaise (gluten-free, if a concern)
- 6 Romaine lettuce leaves, rinsed
- 6 Round tomato slices (¼ inch thick)

Directions:
1. Preheat the air fryer to 350°F .
2. Mix the oil, oregano, thyme, onion powder, salt, and pepper in a small bowl. Spread this mixture all over the eye of round.
3. When the machine is at temperature, set the beef in the basket and air-fry for 30 to 50 minutes (the range depends on the size of the cut), turning the meat twice, until an instant-read meat thermometer inserted into the thickest piece of the meat registers 130°F for rare, 140°F for medium, or 150°F for well-done.
4. Use kitchen tongs to transfer the beef to a cutting board. Cool for 10 minutes. If serving now, carve into ⅛-inch-thick slices. Spread each roll with 2 tablespoons mayonnaise and divide the beef slices between the rolls. Top with a lettuce leaf and a tomato slice and serve. Or set the beef in a container, cover, and refrigerate for up to 3 days to make cold roast beef sandwiches anytime.

Black Bean Veggie Burgers

Servings: 3
Cooking Time: 10 Minutes
Ingredients:
- 1 cup Drained and rinsed canned black beans
- ⅓ cup Pecan pieces
- ⅓ cup Rolled oats (not quick-cooking or steel-cut; gluten-free, if a concern)
- 2 tablespoons (or 1 small egg) Pasteurized egg substitute, such as Egg Beaters (gluten-free, if a concern)
- 2 teaspoons Red ketchup-like chili sauce, such as Heinz
- ¼ teaspoon Ground cumin
- ¼ teaspoon Dried oregano
- ¼ teaspoon Table salt
- ¼ teaspoon Ground black pepper
- Olive oil
- Olive oil spray

Directions:
1. Preheat the air fryer to 400°F.
2. Put the beans, pecans, oats, egg substitute or egg, chili sauce, cumin, oregano, salt, and pepper in a food processor. Cover and process to a coarse paste that will hold its shape like sugar-cookie dough, adding olive oil in 1-teaspoon increments to get the mixture to blend smoothly. The amount of olive oil is actually dependent on the internal moisture content of the beans and the oats. Figure on about 1 tablespoon (three 1-teaspoon additions) for the smaller batch, with proportional increases for the other batches. A

little too much olive oil can't hurt, but a dry paste will fall apart as it cooks and a far-too-wet paste will stick to the basket.

3. Scrape down and remove the blade. Using clean, wet hands, form the paste into two 4-inch patties for the small batch, three 4-inch patties for the medium, or four 4-inch patties for the large batch, setting them one by one on a cutting board. Generously coat both sides of the patties with olive oil spray.

4. Set them in the basket in one layer. Air-fry undisturbed for 10 minutes, or until lightly browned and crisp at the edges.

5. Use a nonstick-safe spatula, and perhaps a flatware fork for balance, to transfer the burgers to a wire rack. Cool for 5 minutes before serving.

Asian Glazed Meatballs

Servings: 4

Cooking Time: 10 Minutes

Ingredients:

- 1 large shallot, finely chopped
- 2 cloves garlic, minced
- 1 tablespoon grated fresh ginger
- 2 teaspoons fresh thyme, finely chopped
- 1½ cups brown mushrooms, very finely chopped (a food processor works well here)
- 2 tablespoons soy sauce
- freshly ground black pepper
- 1 pound ground beef
- ½ pound ground pork
- 3 egg yolks
- 1 cup Thai sweet chili sauce (spring roll sauce)
- ¼ cup toasted sesame seeds
- 2 scallions, sliced

Directions:

1. Combine the shallot, garlic, ginger, thyme, mushrooms, soy sauce, freshly ground black

pepper, ground beef and pork, and egg yolks in a bowl and mix the ingredients together. Gently shape the mixture into 24 balls, about the size of a golf ball.

2. Preheat the air fryer to 380°F.

3. Working in batches, air-fry the meatballs for 8 minutes, turning the meatballs over halfway through the cooking time. Drizzle some of the Thai sweet chili sauce on top of each meatball and return the basket to the air fryer, air-frying for another 2 minutes. Reserve the remaining Thai sweet chili sauce for serving.

4. As soon as the meatballs are done, sprinkle with toasted sesame seeds and transfer them to a serving platter. Scatter the scallions around and serve warm.

Turkey Burgers

Servings: 3

Cooking Time: 23 Minutes

Ingredients:

- 1 pound 2 ounces Ground turkey
- 6 tablespoons Frozen chopped spinach, thawed and squeezed dry
- 3 tablespoons Plain panko bread crumbs (gluten-free, if a concern)
- 1 tablespoon Dijon mustard (gluten-free, if a concern)
- 1½ teaspoons Minced garlic
- ¾ teaspoon Table salt
- ¾ teaspoon Ground black pepper
- Olive oil spray
- 3 Kaiser rolls (gluten-free, if a concern), split open

Directions:

1. Preheat the air fryer to 375°F .

2. Gently mix the ground turkey, spinach, bread crumbs, mustard, garlic, salt, and pepper in a

large bowl until well combined, trying to keep some of the fibers of the ground turkey intact. Form into two 5-inch-wide patties for the small batch, three 5-inch patties for the medium batch, or four 5-inch patties for the large. Coat each side of the patties with olive oil spray.

3. Set the patties in in the basket in one layer and air-fry undisturbed for 20 minutes, or until an instant-read meat thermometer inserted into the center of a burger registers 165°F. You may need to add 2 minutes to the cooking time if the air fryer is at 360°F.

4. Use a nonstick-safe spatula, and perhaps a flatware fork for balance, to transfer the burgers to a cutting board. Set the buns cut side down in the basket in one layer (working in batches as necessary) and air-fry for 1 minute, to toast a bit and warm up. Serve the burgers warm in the buns.

White Bean Veggie Burgers

Servings: 3
Cooking Time: 13 Minutes
Ingredients:
- 1⅓ cups Drained and rinsed canned white beans
- 3 tablespoons Rolled oats (not quick-cooking or steel-cut; gluten-free, if a concern)
- 3 tablespoons Chopped walnuts
- 2 teaspoons Olive oil
- 2 teaspoons Lemon juice
- 1½ teaspoons Dijon mustard (gluten-free, if a concern)
- ¾ teaspoon Dried sage leaves
- ¼ teaspoon Table salt
- Olive oil spray
- 3 Whole-wheat buns or gluten-free whole-grain buns (if a concern), split open

Directions:

1. Preheat the air fryer to 400°F.

2. Place the beans, oats, walnuts, oil, lemon juice, mustard, sage, and salt in a food processor. Cover and process to make a coarse paste that will hold its shape, about like wet sugar-cookie dough, stopping the machine to scrape down the inside of the canister at least once.

3. Scrape down and remove the blade. With clean and wet hands, form the bean paste into two 4-inch patties for the small batch, three 4-inch patties for the medium, or four 4-inch patties for the large batch. Generously coat the patties on both sides with olive oil spray.

4. Set them in the basket with some space between them and air-fry undisturbed for 12 minutes, or until lightly brown and crisp at the edges. The tops of the burgers will feel firm to the touch.

5. Use a nonstick-safe spatula, and perhaps a flatware fork for balance, to transfer the burgers to a cutting board. Set the buns cut side down in the basket in one layer (working in batches as necessary) and air-fry undisturbed for 1 minute, to toast a bit and warm up. Serve the burgers warm in the buns.

Chicken Apple Brie Melt

Servings: 3
Cooking Time: 13 Minutes
Ingredients:
- 3 5- to 6-ounce boneless skinless chicken breasts
- Vegetable oil spray
- 1½ teaspoons Dried herbes de Provence
- 3 ounces Brie, rind removed, thinly sliced
- 6 Thin cored apple slices
- 3 French rolls (gluten-free, if a concern)

- 2 tablespoons Dijon mustard (gluten-free, if a concern)

Directions:

1. Preheat the air fryer to 375°F .
2. Lightly coat all sides of the chicken breasts with vegetable oil spray. Sprinkle the breasts evenly with the herbes de Provence.
3. When the machine is at temperature, set the breasts in the basket and air-fry undisturbed for 10 minutes.
4. Top the chicken breasts with the apple slices, then the cheese. Air-fry undisturbed for 2 minutes, or until the cheese is melty and bubbling.
5. Use a nonstick-safe spatula and kitchen tongs, for balance, to transfer the breasts to a cutting board. Set the rolls in the basket and air-fry for 1 minute to warm through. (Putting them in the machine without splitting them keeps the insides very soft while the outside gets a little crunchy.)
6. Transfer the rolls to the cutting board. Split them open lengthwise, then spread 1 teaspoon mustard on each cut side. Set a prepared chicken breast on the bottom of a roll and close with its top, repeating as necessary to make additional sandwiches. Serve warm.

Chicken Spiedies

Servings: 3
Cooking Time: 12 Minutes

Ingredients:

- 1¼ pounds Boneless skinless chicken thighs, trimmed of any fat blobs and cut into 2-inch pieces
- 3 tablespoons Red wine vinegar
- 2 tablespoons Olive oil
- 2 tablespoons Minced fresh mint leaves
- 2 tablespoons Minced fresh parsley leaves
- 2 teaspoons Minced fresh dill fronds
- ¾ teaspoon Fennel seeds
- ¾ teaspoon Table salt
- Up to a ¼ teaspoon Red pepper flakes
- 3 Long soft rolls, such as hero, hoagie, or Italian sub rolls (gluten-free, if a concern), split open lengthwise
- 4½ tablespoons Regular or low-fat mayonnaise (not fat-free; gluten-free, if a concern)
- 1½ tablespoons Distilled white vinegar
- 1½ teaspoons Ground black pepper

Directions:

1. Mix the chicken, vinegar, oil, mint, parsley, dill, fennel seeds, salt, and red pepper flakes in a zip-closed plastic bag. Seal, gently massage the marinade ingredients into the meat, and refrigerate for at least 2 hours or up to 6 hours. (Longer than that and the meat can turn rubbery.)
2. Set the plastic bag out on the counter (to make the contents a little less frigid). Preheat the air fryer to 400°F.
3. When the machine is at temperature, use kitchen tongs to set the chicken thighs in the basket (discard any remaining marinade) and air-fry undisturbed for 6 minutes. Turn the thighs over and continue air-frying undisturbed for 6 minutes more, until well browned, cooked through, and even a little crunchy.
4. Dump the contents of the basket onto a wire rack and cool for 2 or 3 minutes. Divide the chicken evenly between the rolls. Whisk the mayonnaise, vinegar, and black pepper in a small bowl until smooth. Drizzle this sauce over the chicken pieces in the rolls.

Thai-style Pork Sliders

Servings: 4
Cooking Time: 15 Minutes

Ingredients:

- 11 ounces Ground pork
- 2½ tablespoons Very thinly sliced scallions, white and green parts
- 4 teaspoons Minced peeled fresh ginger
- 2½ teaspoons Fish sauce (gluten-free, if a concern)
- 2 teaspoons Thai curry paste (see the headnote; gluten-free, if a concern)
- 2 teaspoons Light brown sugar
- ¾ teaspoon Ground black pepper
- 4 Slider buns (gluten-free, if a concern)

Directions:

1. Preheat the air fryer to 375°F .

2. Gently mix the pork, scallions, ginger, fish sauce, curry paste, brown sugar, and black pepper in a bowl until well combined. With clean, wet hands, form about ⅓ cup of the pork mixture into a slider about 2½ inches in diameter. Repeat until you use up all the meat—3 sliders for the small batch, 4 for the medium, and 6 for the large. (Keep wetting your hands to help the patties adhere.)

3. When the machine is at temperature, set the sliders in the basket in one layer. Air-fry undisturbed for 14 minutes, or until the sliders are golden brown and caramelized at their edges and an instant-read meat thermometer inserted into the center of a slider registers 160°F.

4. Use a nonstick-safe spatula, and perhaps a flatware fork for balance, to transfer the sliders to a cutting board. Set the buns cut side down in the basket in one layer (working in batches as necessary) and air-fry undisturbed for 1 minute, to toast a bit and warm up. Serve the sliders warm in the buns.

Perfect Burgers

Servings: 3

Cooking Time: 13 Minutes

Ingredients:

- 1 pound 2 ounces 90% lean ground beef
- 1½ tablespoons Worcestershire sauce (gluten-free, if a concern)
- ½ teaspoon Ground black pepper
- 3 Hamburger buns (gluten-free if a concern), split open

Directions:

1. Preheat the air fryer to 375°F .

2. Gently mix the ground beef, Worcestershire sauce, and pepper in a bowl until well combined but preserving as much of the meat's fibers as possible. Divide this mixture into two 5-inch patties for the small batch, three 5-inch patties for the medium, or four 5-inch patties for the large. Make a thumbprint indentation in the center of each patty, about halfway through the meat.

3. Set the patties in the basket in one layer with some space between them. Air-fry undisturbed for 10 minutes, or until an instant-read meat thermometer inserted into the center of a burger registers 160°F (a medium-well burger). You may need to add 2 minutes cooking time if the air fryer is at 360°F.

4. Use a nonstick-safe spatula, and perhaps a flatware fork for balance, to transfer the burgers to a cutting board. Set the buns cut side down in the basket in one layer (working in batches as necessary) and air-fry undisturbed for 1 minute, to toast a bit and warm up. Serve the burgers in the warm buns.

Sausage And Pepper Heros

Servings: 3
Cooking Time: 11 Minutes
Ingredients:

- 3 links (about 9 ounces total) Sweet Italian sausages (gluten-free, if a concern)
- 1½ Medium red or green bell pepper(s), stemmed, cored, and cut into ½-inch-wide strips
- 1 medium Yellow or white onion(s), peeled, halved, and sliced into thin half-moons
- 3 Long soft rolls, such as hero, hoagie, or Italian sub rolls (gluten-free, if a concern), split open lengthwise
- For garnishing Balsamic vinegar
- For garnishing Fresh basil leaves

Directions:

1. Preheat the air fryer to 400°F.

2. When the machine is at temperature, set the sausage links in the basket in one layer and air-fry undisturbed for 5 minutes.

3. Add the pepper strips and onions. Continue air-frying, tossing and rearranging everything about once every minute, for 5 minutes, or until the sausages are browned and an instant-read meat thermometer inserted into one of the links registers 160°F.

4. Use a nonstick-safe spatula and kitchen tongs to transfer the sausages and vegetables to a cutting board. Set the rolls cut side down in the basket in one layer (working in batches as necessary) and air-fry undisturbed for 1 minute, to toast the rolls a bit and warm them up. Set 1 sausage with some pepper strips and onions in each warm roll, sprinkle balsamic vinegar over the sandwich fillings, and garnish with basil leaves.

Dijon Thyme Burgers

Servings: 3
Cooking Time: 18 Minutes

Ingredients:

- 1 pound lean ground beef
- ⅓ cup panko breadcrumbs
- ¼ cup finely chopped onion
- 3 tablespoons Dijon mustard
- 1 tablespoon chopped fresh thyme
- 4 teaspoons Worcestershire sauce
- 1 teaspoon salt
- freshly ground black pepper
- Topping (optional):
- 2 tablespoons Dijon mustard
- 1 tablespoon dark brown sugar
- 1 teaspoon Worcestershire sauce
- 4 ounces sliced Swiss cheese, optional

Directions:

1. Combine all the burger ingredients together in a large bowl and mix well. Divide the meat into 4 equal portions and then form the burgers, being careful not to over-handle the meat. One good way to do this is to throw the meat back and forth from one hand to another, packing the meat each time you catch it. Flatten the balls into patties, making an indentation in the center of each patty with your thumb (this will help it stay flat as it cooks) and flattening the sides of the burgers so that they will fit nicely into the air fryer basket.

2. Preheat the air fryer to 370°F.

3. If you don't have room for all four burgers, air-fry two or three burgers at a time for 8 minutes. Flip the burgers over and air-fry for another 6 minutes.

4. While the burgers are cooking combine the Dijon mustard, dark brown sugar, and Worcestershire sauce in a small bowl and mix well. This optional topping to the burgers really adds a boost of flavor at the end. Spread the Dijon topping evenly on each burger. If you cooked the burgers in batches, return the first batch to the cooker at this time – it's ok to place the fourth burger on top of the others in the

center of the basket. Air-fry the burgers for another 3 minutes.

5. Finally, if desired, top each burger with a slice of Swiss cheese. Lower the air fryer temperature to 330°F and air-fry for another minute to melt the cheese. Serve the burgers on toasted brioche buns, dressed the way you like them.

Thanksgiving Turkey Sandwiches

Servings: 3

Cooking Time: 10 Minutes

Ingredients:

- 1½ cups Herb-seasoned stuffing mix (not cornbread-style; gluten-free, if a concern)
- 1 Large egg white(s)
- 2 tablespoons Water
- 3 5- to 6-ounce turkey breast cutlets
- Vegetable oil spray
- 4½ tablespoons Purchased cranberry sauce, preferably whole berry
- ⅛ teaspoon Ground cinnamon
- ⅛ teaspoon Ground dried ginger
- 4½ tablespoons Regular, low-fat, or fat-free mayonnaise (gluten-free, if a concern)
- 6 tablespoons Shredded Brussels sprouts
- 3 Kaiser rolls (gluten-free, if a concern), split open

Directions:

1. Preheat the air fryer to 375°F .

2. Put the stuffing mix in a heavy zip-closed bag, seal it, lay it flat on your counter, and roll a rolling pin over the bag to crush the stuffing mix to the consistency of rough sand. (Or you can pulse the stuffing mix to the desired consistency in a food processor.)

3. Set up and fill two shallow soup plates or small pie plates on your counter: one for the egg white(s), whisked with the water until foamy; and one for the ground stuffing mix.

4. Dip a cutlet in the egg white mixture, coating both sides and letting any excess egg white slip back into the rest. Set the cutlet in the ground stuffing mix and coat it evenly on both sides, pressing gently to coat well on both sides. Lightly coat the cutlet on both sides with vegetable oil spray, set it aside, and continue dipping and coating the remaining cutlets in the same way.

5. Set the cutlets in the basket and air-fry undisturbed for 10 minutes, or until crisp and brown. Use kitchen tongs to transfer the cutlets to a wire rack to cool for a few minutes.

6. Meanwhile, stir the cranberry sauce with the cinnamon and ginger in a small bowl. Mix the shredded Brussels sprouts and mayonnaise in a second bowl until the vegetable is evenly coated.

7. Build the sandwiches by spreading about 1½ tablespoons of the cranberry mixture on the cut side of the bottom half of each roll. Set a cutlet on top, then spread about 3 tablespoons of the Brussels sprouts mixture evenly over the cutlet. Set the other half of the roll on top and serve warm.

Lamb Burgers

Servings: 3

Cooking Time: 17 Minutes

Ingredients:

- 1 pound 2 ounces Ground lamb
- 3 tablespoons Crumbled feta
- 1 teaspoon Minced garlic
- 1 teaspoon Tomato paste
- ¾ teaspoon Ground coriander
- ¾ teaspoon Ground dried ginger
- Up to ⅛ teaspoon Cayenne
- Up to a ⅛ teaspoon Table salt (optional)
- 3 Kaiser rolls or hamburger buns (gluten-free, if a concern), split open

Directions:

1. Preheat the air fryer to 375°F .

2. Gently mix the ground lamb, feta, garlic, tomato paste, coriander, ginger, cayenne, and salt (if using) in a bowl until well combined, trying to keep the bits of cheese intact. Form this mixture into two 5-inch patties for the small batch, three 5-inch patties for the medium, or four 5-inch patties for the large.

3. Set the patties in the basket in one layer and air-fry undisturbed for 16 minutes, or until an instant-read meat thermometer inserted into one burger registers 160°F. (The cheese is not an issue with the temperature probe in this recipe as it was for the Inside-Out Cheeseburgers, because the feta is so well mixed into the ground meat.)

4. Use a nonstick-safe spatula, and perhaps a flatware fork for balance, to transfer the burgers to a cutting board. Set the buns cut side down in the basket in one layer (working in batches as necessary) and air-fry undisturbed for 1 minute, to toast a bit and warm up. Serve the burgers warm in the buns.

Chicken Club Sandwiches

Servings: 3

Cooking Time: 15 Minutes

Ingredients:

- 3 5- to 6-ounce boneless skinless chicken breasts
- 6 Thick-cut bacon strips (gluten-free, if a concern)
- 3 Long soft rolls, such as hero, hoagie, or Italian sub rolls (gluten-free, if a concern)
- 3 tablespoons Regular, low-fat, or fat-free mayonnaise (gluten-free, if a concern)
- 3 Lettuce leaves, preferably romaine or iceberg
- 6 ¼-inch-thick tomato slices

Directions:

1. Preheat the air fryer to 375°F .

2. Wrap each chicken breast with 2 strips of bacon, spiraling the bacon around the meat, slightly overlapping the strips on each revolution. Start the second strip of bacon farther down the breast but on a line with the start of the first strip so they both end at a lined-up point on the chicken breast.

3. When the machine is at temperature, set the wrapped breasts bacon-seam side down in the basket with space between them. Air-fry undisturbed for 12 minutes, until the bacon is browned, crisp, and cooked through and an instant-read meat thermometer inserted into the center of a breast registers 165°F. You may need to add 2 minutes in the air fryer if the temperature is at 360°F.

4. Use kitchen tongs to transfer the breasts to a wire rack. Split the rolls open lengthwise and set them cut side down in the basket. Air-fry for 1 minute, or until warmed through.

5. Use kitchen tongs to transfer the rolls to a cutting board. Spread 1 tablespoon mayonnaise on the cut side of one half of each roll. Top with a chicken breast, lettuce leaf, and tomato slice. Serve warm.

Inside-out Cheeseburgers

Servings: 3
Cooking Time: 9-11 Minutes
Ingredients:
- 1 pound 2 ounces 90% lean ground beef
- ¾ teaspoon Dried oregano
- ¾ teaspoon Table salt
- ¾ teaspoon Ground black pepper
- ¼ teaspoon Garlic powder
- 6 tablespoons (about 1½ ounces) Shredded Cheddar, Swiss, or other semi-firm cheese, or a purchased blend of shredded cheeses
- 3 Hamburger buns (gluten-free, if a concern), split open

Directions:
1. Preheat the air fryer to 375°F .
2. Gently mix the ground beef, oregano, salt, pepper, and garlic powder in a bowl until well combined without turning the mixture to mush. Form it into two 6-inch patties for the small batch, three for the medium, or four for the large.
3. Place 2 tablespoons of the shredded cheese in the center of each patty. With clean hands, fold the sides of the patty up to cover the cheese, then pick it up and roll it gently into a ball to seal the cheese inside. Gently press it back into a 5-inch burger without letting any cheese squish out. Continue filling and preparing more burgers, as needed.
4. Place the burgers in the basket in one layer and air-fry undisturbed for 8 minutes for medium or 10 minutes for well-done. (An instant-read meat thermometer won't work for these burgers because it will hit the mostly melted cheese inside and offer a hotter temperature than the surrounding meat.)
5. Use a nonstick-safe spatula, and perhaps a flatware fork for balance, to transfer the burgers to a cutting board. Set the buns cut side down in the basket in one layer (working in batches as necessary) and air-fry undisturbed for 1 minute, to toast a bit and warm up. Cool the burgers a few minutes more, then serve them warm in the buns.

Provolone Stuffed Meatballs

Servings: 4
Cooking Time: 12 Minutes
Ingredients:
- 1 tablespoon olive oil
- 1 small onion, very finely chopped
- 1 to 2 cloves garlic, minced
- ¾ pound ground beef
- ¾ pound ground pork
- ¾ cup breadcrumbs
- ¼ cup grated Parmesan cheese
- ¼ cup finely chopped fresh parsley (or 1 tablespoon dried parsley)
- ½ teaspoon dried oregano
- 1½ teaspoons salt
- freshly ground black pepper
- 2 eggs, lightly beaten
- 5 ounces sharp or aged provolone cheese, cut into 1-inch cubes

Directions:
1. Preheat a skillet over medium-high heat. Add the oil and cook the onion and garlic until tender, but not browned.
2. Transfer the onion and garlic to a large bowl and add the beef, pork, breadcrumbs, Parmesan

cheese, parsley, oregano, salt, pepper and eggs. Mix well until all the ingredients are combined. Divide the mixture into 12 evenly sized balls. Make one meatball at a time, by pressing a hole in the meatball mixture with your finger and pushing a piece of provolone cheese into the hole. Mold the meat back into a ball, enclosing the cheese.

3. Preheat the air fryer to 380°F.

4. Working in two batches, transfer six of the meatballs to the air fryer basket and air-fry for 12 minutes, shaking the basket and turning the meatballs a couple of times during the cooking process. Repeat with the remaining six meatballs. You can pop the first batch of meatballs into the air fryer for the last two minutes of cooking to re-heat them. Serve warm.

Chicken Gyros

Servings: 4
Cooking Time: 14 Minutes
Ingredients:
- 4 4- to 5-ounce boneless skinless chicken thighs, trimmed of any fat blobs
- 2 tablespoons Lemon juice
- 2 tablespoons Red wine vinegar
- 2 tablespoons Olive oil
- 2 teaspoons Dried oregano
- 2 teaspoons Minced garlic
- 1 teaspoon Table salt
- 1 teaspoon Ground black pepper
- 4 Pita pockets (gluten-free, if a concern)
- ½ cup Chopped tomatoes
- ½ cup Bottled regular, low-fat, or fat-free ranch dressing (gluten-free, if a concern)

Directions:
1. Mix the thighs, lemon juice, vinegar, oil, oregano, garlic, salt, and pepper in a zip-closed bag. Seal, gently massage the marinade into the meat through the plastic, and refrigerate for at least 2 hours or up to 6 hours. (Longer than that and the meat can turn rubbery.)

2. Set the plastic bag out on the counter (to make the contents a little less frigid). Preheat the air fryer to 375°F .

3. When the machine is at temperature, use kitchen tongs to place the thighs in the basket in one layer. Discard the marinade. Air-fry the chicken thighs undisturbed for 12 minutes, or until browned and an instant-read meat thermometer inserted into the thickest part of one thigh registers 165°F. You may need to air-fry the chicken 2 minutes longer if the machine's temperature is 360°F.

4. Use kitchen tongs to transfer the thighs to a cutting board. Cool for 5 minutes, then set one thigh in each of the pita pockets. Top each with 2 tablespoons chopped tomatoes and 2 tablespoons dressing. Serve warm.

Philly Cheesesteak Sandwiches

Servings: 3
Cooking Time: 9 Minutes
Ingredients:
- ¾ pound Shaved beef
- 1 tablespoon Worcestershire sauce (gluten-free, if a concern)
- ¼ teaspoon Garlic powder
- ¼ teaspoon Mild paprika
- 6 tablespoons (1½ ounces) Frozen bell pepper strips (do not thaw)
- 2 slices, broken into rings Very thin yellow or white medium onion slice(s)
- 6 ounces (6 to 8 slices) Provolone cheese slices

• 3 Long soft rolls such as hero, hoagie, or Italian sub rolls, or hot dog buns (gluten-free, if a concern), split open lengthwise

Directions:

1. Preheat the air fryer to 400°F.

2. When the machine is at temperature, spread the shaved beef in the basket, leaving a ½-inch perimeter around the meat for good air flow. Sprinkle the meat with the Worcestershire sauce, paprika, and garlic powder. Spread the peppers and onions on top of the meat.

3. Air-fry undisturbed for 6 minutes, or until cooked through. Set the cheese on top of the meat. Continue air-frying undisturbed for 3 minutes, or until the cheese has melted.

4. Use kitchen tongs to divide the meat and cheese layers in the basket between the rolls or buns. Serve hot.

Eggplant Parmesan Subs

Servings: 2
Cooking Time: 13 Minutes

Ingredients:

• 4 Peeled eggplant slices (about ½ inch thick and 3 inches in diameter)

• Olive oil spray

• 2 tablespoons plus 2 teaspoons Jarred pizza sauce, any variety except creamy

• ¼ cup (about ⅔ ounce) Finely grated Parmesan cheese

• 2 Small, long soft rolls, such as hero, hoagie, or Italian sub rolls (gluten-free, if a concern), split open lengthwise

Directions:

1. Preheat the air fryer to 350°F .

2. When the machine is at temperature, coat both sides of the eggplant slices with olive oil spray. Set them in the basket in one layer and air-

fry undisturbed for 10 minutes, until lightly browned and softened.

3. Increase the machine's temperature to 375°F (or 370°F, if that's the closest setting—unless the machine is already at 360°F, in which case leave it alone). Top each eggplant slice with 2 teaspoons pizza sauce, then 1 tablespoon cheese. Air-fry undisturbed for 2 minutes, or until the cheese has melted.

4. Use a nonstick-safe spatula, and perhaps a flatware fork for balance, to transfer the eggplant slices cheese side up to a cutting board. Set the roll(s) cut side down in the basket in one layer (working in batches as necessary) and air-fry undisturbed for 1 minute, to toast the rolls a bit and warm them up. Set 2 eggplant slices in each warm roll.

Reuben Sandwiches

Servings: 2
Cooking Time: 11 Minutes

Ingredients:

• ½ pound Sliced deli corned beef

• 4 teaspoons Regular or low-fat mayonnaise (not fat-free)

• 4 Rye bread slices

• 2 tablespoons plus 2 teaspoons Russian dressing

• ½ cup Purchased sauerkraut, squeezed by the handful over the sink to get rid of excess moisture

• 2 ounces (2 to 4 slices) Swiss cheese slices (optional)

Directions:

1. Set the corned beef in the basket, slip the basket into the machine, and heat the air fryer to 400°F. Air-fry undisturbed for 3 minutes from the time the basket is put in the machine, just to warm up the meat.

2. Use kitchen tongs to transfer the corned beef to a cutting board. Spread 1 teaspoon mayonnaise on one side of each slice of rye bread, rubbing the mayonnaise into the bread with a small flatware knife.

3. Place the bread slices mayonnaise side down on a cutting board. Spread the Russian dressing over the "dry" side of each slice. For one sandwich, top one slice of bread with the corned beef, sauerkraut, and cheese (if using). For two sandwiches, top two slices of bread each with half of the corned beef, sauerkraut, and cheese (if using). Close the sandwiches with the remaining bread, setting it mayonnaise side up on top.

4. Set the sandwich(es) in the basket and air-fry undisturbed for 8 minutes, or until browned and crunchy.

5. Use a nonstick-safe spatula, and perhaps a flatware fork for balance, to transfer the sandwich(es) to a cutting board. Cool for 2 or 3 minutes before slicing in half and serving.

Inside Out Cheeseburgers

Servings: 2
Cooking Time: 20 Minutes
Ingredients:
- ¾ pound lean ground beef
- 3 tablespoons minced onion
- 4 teaspoons ketchup
- 2 teaspoons yellow mustard
- salt and freshly ground black pepper
- 4 slices of Cheddar cheese, broken into smaller pieces
- 8 hamburger dill pickle chips

Directions:
1. Combine the ground beef, minced onion, ketchup, mustard, salt and pepper in a large bowl. Mix well to thoroughly combine the ingredients. Divide the meat into four equal portions.

2. To make the stuffed burgers, flatten each portion of meat into a thin patty. Place 4 pickle chips and half of the cheese onto the center of two of the patties, leaving a rim around the edge of the patty exposed. Place the remaining two patties on top of the first and press the meat together firmly, sealing the edges tightly. With the burgers on a flat surface, press the sides of the burger with the palm of your hand to create a straight edge. This will help keep the stuffing inside the burger while it cooks.

3. Preheat the air fryer to 370°F.

4. Place the burgers inside the air fryer basket and air-fry for 20 minutes, flipping the burgers over halfway through the cooking time.

5. Serve the cheeseburgers on buns with lettuce and tomato.

Fish And Seafood Recipes

Sesame-crusted Tuna Steaks

Servings:3

Cooking Time: 10-13 Minutes

Ingredients:

- ½ cup Sesame seeds, preferably a blend of white and black
- 1½ tablespoons Toasted sesame oil
- 3 6-ounce skinless tuna steaks

Directions:

1. Preheat the air fryer to 400°F.

2. Pour the sesame seeds on a dinner plate. Use ½ tablespoon of the sesame oil as a rub on both sides and the edges of a tuna steak. Set it in the sesame seeds, then turn it several times, pressing gently, to create an even coating of the seeds, including around the steak's edge. Set aside and continue coating the remaining steak(s).

3. When the machine is at temperature, set the steaks in the basket with as much air space between them as possible. Air-fry undisturbed for 10 minutes for medium-rare (not USDA-approved), or 12 to 13 minutes for cooked through (USDA-approved).

4. Use a nonstick-safe spatula to transfer the steaks to serving plates. Serve hot.

Flounder Fillets

Servings: 4

Cooking Time: 8 Minutes

Ingredients:

- 1 egg white
- 1 tablespoon water
- 1 cup panko breadcrumbs
- 2 tablespoons extra-light virgin olive oil
- 4 4-ounce flounder fillets
- salt and pepper
- oil for misting or cooking spray

Directions:

1. Preheat air fryer to 390°F.

2. Beat together egg white and water in shallow dish.

3. In another shallow dish, mix panko crumbs and oil until well combined and crumbly (best done by hand).

4. Season flounder fillets with salt and pepper to taste. Dip each fillet into egg mixture and then roll in panko crumbs, pressing in crumbs so that fish is nicely coated.

5. Spray air fryer basket with nonstick cooking spray and add fillets. Cook at 390°F for 3minutes.

6. Spray fish fillets but do not turn. Cook 5 minutes longer or until golden brown and crispy. Using a spatula, carefully remove fish from basket and serve.

Coconut Jerk Shrimp

Servings:3

Cooking Time: 8 Minutes

Ingredients:

- 1 Large egg white(s)
- 1 teaspoon Purchased or homemade jerk dried seasoning blend (see the headnote)
- ¾ cup Plain panko bread crumbs (gluten-free, if a concern)
- ¾ cup Unsweetened shredded coconut
- 12 Large shrimp (20–25 per pound), peeled and deveined
- Coconut oil spray

Directions:

1. Preheat the air fryer to 375°F .

2. Whisk the egg white(s) and seasoning blend in a bowl until foamy. Add the shrimp and toss well to coat evenly.

3. Mix the bread crumbs and coconut on a dinner plate until well combined. Use kitchen tongs to pick up a shrimp, letting the excess egg white mixture slip back into the rest. Set the shrimp in the bread-crumb mixture. Turn several times to coat evenly and thoroughly. Set on a cutting board and continue coating the remainder of the shrimp.

4. Lightly coat all the shrimp on both sides with the coconut oil spray. Set them in the basket in one layer with as much space between them as possible. (You can even stand some up along the basket's wall in some models.) Air-fry undisturbed for 6 minutes, or until the coating is lightly browned. If the air fryer is at 360°F, you may need to add 2 minutes to the cooking time.

5. Use clean kitchen tongs to transfer the shrimp to a wire rack. Cool for only a minute or two before serving.

Classic Crab Cakes

Servings:4
Cooking Time: 10 Minutes
Ingredients:
- 10 ounces Lump crabmeat, picked over for shell and cartilage
- 6 tablespoons Plain panko bread crumbs (gluten-free, if a concern)
- 6 tablespoons Chopped drained jarred roasted red peppers
- 4 Medium scallions, trimmed and thinly sliced
- ¼ cup Regular or low-fat mayonnaise (not fat-free; gluten-free, if a concern)
- ¼ teaspoon Dried dill
- ¼ teaspoon Dried thyme
- ¼ teaspoon Onion powder
- ¼ teaspoon Table salt
- ⅛ teaspoon Celery seeds
- Up to ⅛ teaspoon Cayenne
- Vegetable oil spray

Directions:
1. Preheat the air fryer to 400°F.

2. Gently mix the crabmeat, bread crumbs, red pepper, scallion, mayonnaise, dill, thyme, onion powder, salt, celery seeds, and cayenne in a bowl until well combined.

3. Use clean and dry hands to form ½ cup of this mixture into a tightly packed 1-inch-thick, 3- to 4-inch-wide patty. Coat the top and bottom of the patty with vegetable oil spray and set it aside. Continue making 1 more patty for a small batch, 3 more for a medium batch, or 5 more for a larger one, coating them with vegetable oil spray on both sides.

4. Set the patties in one layer in the basket and air-fry undisturbed for 10 minutes, or until lightly browned and cooked through.

5. Use a nonstick-safe spatula to transfer the crab cakes to a serving platter or plates. Wait a couple of minutes before serving.

Curried Sweet-and-spicy Scallops

Servings:3
Cooking Time: 5 Minutes
Ingredients:
- 6 tablespoons Thai sweet chili sauce
- 2 cups (from about 5 cups cereal) Crushed Rice Krispies or other rice-puff cereal
- 2 teaspoons Yellow curry powder, purchased or homemade (see here)
- 1 pound Sea scallops
- Vegetable oil spray

Directions:

1. Preheat the air fryer to 400°F.

2. Set up and fill two shallow soup plates or small pie plates on your counter: one for the chili sauce and one for crumbs, mixed with the curry powder.

3. Dip a scallop into the chili sauce, coating it on all sides. Set it in the cereal mixture and turn several times to coat evenly. Gently shake off any excess and set the scallop on a cutting board. Continue dipping and coating the remaining scallops. Coat them all on all sides with the vegetable oil spray.

4. Set the scallops in the basket with as much air space between them as possible. Air-fry undisturbed for 5 minutes, or until lightly browned and crunchy.

5. Remove the basket. Set aside for 2 minutes to let the coating set up. Then gently pour the contents of the basket onto a platter and serve at once.

Crispy Sweet-and-sour Cod Fillets

Servings:3
Cooking Time: 12 Minutes

Ingredients:

- 1½ cups Plain panko bread crumbs (gluten-free, if a concern)
- 2 tablespoons Regular or low-fat mayonnaise (not fat-free; gluten-free, if a concern)
- ¼ cup Sweet pickle relish
- 3 4- to 5-ounce skinless cod fillets

Directions:

1. Preheat the air fryer to 400°F.

2. Pour the bread crumbs into a shallow soup plate or a small pie plate. Mix the mayonnaise and relish in a small bowl until well combined. Smear this mixture all over the cod fillets. Set them in the crumbs and turn until evenly coated on all sides, even on the ends.

3. Set the coated cod fillets in the basket with as much air space between them as possible. They should not touch. Air-fry undisturbed for 12 minutes, or until browned and crisp.

4. Use a nonstick-safe spatula to transfer the cod pieces to a wire rack. Cool for only a minute or two before serving hot.

Shrimp "scampi"

Servings:4
Cooking Time: 5 Minutes

Ingredients:

- 1½ pounds Large shrimp (20–25 per pound), peeled and deveined
- ¼ cup Olive oil
- 2 tablespoons Minced garlic
- 1 teaspoon Dried oregano
- Up to 1 teaspoon Red pepper flakes
- ½ teaspoon Table salt
- 2 tablespoons White balsamic vinegar (see here)

Directions:

1. Preheat the air fryer to 400°F.

2. Stir the shrimp, olive oil, garlic, oregano, red pepper flakes, and salt in a large bowl until the shrimp are well coated.

3. When the machine is at temperature, transfer the shrimp to the basket. They will overlap and even sit on top of each other. Air-fry for 5 minutes, tossing and rearranging the shrimp twice to make sure the covered surfaces are exposed, until pink and firm.

4. Pour the contents of the basket into a serving bowl. Pour the vinegar over the shrimp while hot and toss to coat.

Crab Stuffed Salmon Roast

Servings: 4
Cooking Time: 20 Minutes
Ingredients:
- 1 (1½-pound) salmon fillet
- salt and freshly ground black pepper
- 6 ounces crabmeat
- 1 teaspoon finely chopped lemon zest
- 1 teaspoon Dijon mustard
- 1 tablespoon chopped fresh parsley, plus more for garnish
- 1 scallion, chopped
- ¼ teaspoon salt
- olive oil

Directions:
1. Prepare the salmon fillet by butterflying it. Slice into the thickest side of the salmon, parallel to the countertop and along the length of the fillet. Don't slice all the way through to the other side – stop about an inch from the edge. Open the salmon up like a book. Season the salmon with salt and freshly ground black pepper.
2. Make the crab filling by combining the crabmeat, lemon zest, mustard, parsley, scallion, salt and freshly ground black pepper in a bowl. Spread this filling in the center of the salmon. Fold one side of the salmon over the filling. Then fold the other side over on top.
3. Transfer the rolled salmon to the center of a piece of parchment paper that is roughly 6- to 7-inches wide and about 12-inches long. The parchment paper will act as a sling, making it easier to put the salmon into the air fryer. Preheat the air fryer to 370°F. Use the parchment paper to transfer the salmon roast to the air fryer basket and tuck the ends of the paper down beside the salmon. Drizzle a little olive oil on top and season with salt and pepper.
4. Air-fry the salmon at 370°F for 20 minutes.
5. Remove the roast from the air fryer and let it rest for a few minutes. Then, slice it, sprinkle some more lemon zest and parsley (or fresh chives) on top and serve.

Nutty Shrimp With Amaretto Glaze

Servings: 10
Cooking Time: 10 Minutes
Ingredients:
- 1 cup flour
- ½ teaspoon baking powder
- 1 teaspoon salt
- 2 eggs, beaten
- ½ cup milk
- 2 tablespoons olive or vegetable oil
- 2 cups sliced almonds
- 2 pounds large shrimp (about 32 to 40 shrimp), peeled and deveined, tails left on
- 2 cups amaretto liqueur

Directions:
1. Combine the flour, baking powder and salt in a large bowl. Add the eggs, milk and oil and stir until it forms a smooth batter. Coarsely crush the sliced almonds into a second shallow dish with your hands.
2. Dry the shrimp well with paper towels. Dip the shrimp into the batter and shake off any excess batter, leaving just enough to lightly coat the shrimp. Transfer the shrimp to the dish with the almonds and coat completely. Place the coated shrimp on a plate or baking sheet and when all the shrimp have been coated, freeze the shrimp for an 1 hour, or as long as a week before air-frying.
3. Preheat the air fryer to 400°F.

4. Transfer 8 frozen shrimp at a time to the air fryer basket. Air-fry for 6 minutes. Turn the shrimp over and air-fry for an additional 4 minutes. Repeat with the remaining shrimp.

5. While the shrimp are cooking, bring the Amaretto to a boil in a small saucepan on the stovetop. Lower the heat and simmer until it has reduced and thickened into a glaze – about 10 minutes.

6. Remove the shrimp from the air fryer and brush both sides with the warm amaretto glaze. Serve warm.

Pecan-crusted Tilapia

Servings: 4

Cooking Time: 8 Minutes

Ingredients:
- 1 pound skinless, boneless tilapia filets
- ¼ cup butter, melted
- 1 teaspoon minced fresh or dried rosemary
- 1 cup finely chopped pecans
- 1 teaspoon sea salt
- ¼ teaspoon paprika
- 2 tablespoons chopped parsley
- 1 lemon, cut into wedges

Directions:

1. Pat the tilapia filets dry with paper towels.

2. Pour the melted butter over the filets and flip the filets to coat them completely.

3. In a medium bowl, mix together the rosemary, pecans, salt, and paprika.

4. Preheat the air fryer to 350°F.

5. Place the tilapia filets into the air fryer basket and top with the pecan coating. Cook for 6 to 8 minutes. The fish should be firm to the touch and flake easily when fully cooked.

6. Remove the fish from the air fryer. Top the fish with chopped parsley and serve with lemon wedges.

Fried Shrimp

Servings:3

Cooking Time: 7 Minutes

Ingredients:
- 1 Large egg white
- 2 tablespoons Water
- 1 cup Plain dried bread crumbs (gluten-free, if a concern)
- ¼ cup All-purpose flour or almond flour
- ¼ cup Yellow cornmeal
- 1 teaspoon Celery salt
- 1 teaspoon Mild paprika
- Up to ½ teaspoon Cayenne (optional)
- ¾ pound Large shrimp (20–25 per pound), peeled and deveined
- Vegetable oil spray

Directions:

1. Preheat the air fryer to 400°F.

2. Set two medium or large bowls on your counter. In the first, whisk the egg white and water until foamy. In the second, stir the bread crumbs, flour, cornmeal, celery salt, paprika, and cayenne (if using) until well combined.

3. Pour all the shrimp into the egg white mixture and stir gently until all the shrimp are coated. Use kitchen tongs to pick them up one by one and transfer them to the bread-crumb mixture. Turn each in the bread-crumb mixture to coat it evenly and thoroughly on all sides before setting it on a cutting board. When you're done coating the shrimp, coat them all on both sides with the vegetable oil spray.

4. Set the shrimp in as close to one layer in the basket as you can. Some may overlap. Air-fry for

7 minutes, gently rearranging the shrimp at the 4-minute mark to get covered surfaces exposed, until golden brown and firm but not hard.

5. Use kitchen tongs to gently transfer the shrimp to a wire rack. Cool for only a minute or two before serving.

Buttery Lobster Tails

Servings:4

Cooking Time: 6 Minutes

Ingredients:

- 4 6- to 8-ounce shell-on raw lobster tails
- 2 tablespoons Butter, melted and cooled
- 1 teaspoon Lemon juice
- ½ teaspoon Finely grated lemon zest
- ½ teaspoon Garlic powder
- ½ teaspoon Table salt
- ½ teaspoon Ground black pepper

Directions:

1. Preheat the air fryer to 375°F .

2. To give the tails that restaurant look, you need to butterfly the meat. To do so, place a tail on a cutting board so that the shell is convex. Use kitchen shears to cut a line down the middle of the shell from the larger end to the smaller, cutting only the shell and not the meat below, and stopping before the back fins. Pry open the shell, leaving it intact. Use your clean fingers to separate the meat from the shell's sides and bottom, keeping it attached to the shell at the back near the fins. Pull the meat up and out of the shell through the cut line, laying the meat on top of the shell and closing the shell (as well as you can) under the meat. Make two equidistant cuts down the meat from the larger end to near the smaller end, each about ¼ inch deep, for the classic restaurant look on the plate. Repeat this procedure with the remaining tail(s).

3. Stir the butter, lemon juice, zest, garlic powder, salt, and pepper in a small bowl until well combined. Brush this mixture over the lobster meat set atop the shells.

4. When the machine is at temperature, place the tails shell side down in the basket with as much air space between them as possible. Air-fry undisturbed for 6 minutes, or until the lobster meat has pink streaks over it and is firm.

5. Use kitchen tongs to transfer the tails to a wire rack. Cool for only a minute or two before serving.

Lightened-up Breaded Fish Filets

Servings: 4

Cooking Time: 10 Minutes

Ingredients:

- ½ cup all-purpose flour
- ½ teaspoon cayenne pepper
- 1 teaspoon garlic powder
- ½ teaspoon black pepper
- ¼ teaspoon salt
- 2 eggs, whisked
- 1½ cups panko breadcrumbs
- 1 pound boneless white fish filets
- 1 cup tartar sauce
- 1 lemon, sliced into wedges

Directions:

1. In a medium bowl, mix the flour, cayenne pepper, garlic powder, pepper, and salt.

2. In a shallow dish, place the eggs.

3. In a third dish, place the breadcrumbs.

4. Cover the fish in the flour, dip them in the egg, and coat them with panko. Repeat until all fish are covered in the breading.

5. Liberally spray the metal trivet that fits inside the air fryer basket with olive oil mist. Place the fish onto the trivet, leaving space between the

filets to flip. Cook for 5 minutes, flip the fish, and cook another 5 minutes. Repeat until all the fish is cooked.

6. Serve warm with tartar sauce and lemon wedges.

Five Spice Red Snapper With Green Onions And Orange Salsa

Servings: 2
Cooking Time: 8 Minutes
Ingredients:
- 2 oranges, peeled, segmented and chopped
- 1 tablespoon minced shallot
- 1 to 3 teaspoons minced red Jalapeño or Serrano pepper
- 1 tablespoon chopped fresh cilantro
- lime juice, to taste
- salt, to taste
- 2 (5- to 6-ounce) red snapper fillets
- ½ teaspoon Chinese five spice powder
- salt and freshly ground black pepper
- vegetable or olive oil, in a spray bottle
- 4 green onions, cut into 2-inch lengths

Directions:
1. Start by making the salsa. Cut the peel off the oranges, slicing around the oranges to expose the flesh. Segment the oranges by cutting in between the membranes of the orange. Chop the segments roughly and combine in a bowl with the shallot, Jalapeño or Serrano pepper, cilantro, lime juice and salt. Set the salsa aside.
2. Preheat the air fryer to 400°F.
3. Season the fish fillets with the five-spice powder, salt and freshly ground black pepper. Spray both sides of the fish fillets with oil. Toss the green onions with a little oil.
4. Transfer the fish to the air fryer basket and scatter the green onions around the fish. Air-fry at 400°F for 8 minutes.

5. Remove the fish from the air fryer, along with the fried green onions. Serve with white rice and a spoonful of the salsa on top.

Crab Cakes On A Budget

Servings: 4
Cooking Time: 12 Minutes
Ingredients:
- 8 ounces imitation crabmeat
- 4 ounces leftover cooked fish (such as cod, pollock, or haddock)
- 2 tablespoons minced green onion
- 2 tablespoons minced celery
- ¾ cup crushed saltine cracker crumbs
- 2 tablespoons light mayonnaise
- 1 teaspoon prepared yellow mustard
- 1 tablespoon Worcestershire sauce, plus 2 teaspoons
- 2 teaspoons dried parsley flakes
- ½ teaspoon dried dill weed, crushed
- ½ teaspoon garlic powder
- ½ teaspoon Old Bay Seasoning
- ½ cup panko breadcrumbs
- oil for misting or cooking spray

Directions:
1. Use knives or a food processor to finely shred crabmeat and fish.
2. In a large bowl, combine all ingredients except panko and oil. Stir well.
3. Shape into 8 small, fat patties.
4. Carefully roll patties in panko crumbs to coat. Spray both sides with oil or cooking spray.
5. Place patties in air fryer basket and cook at 390°F for 12 minutes or until golden brown and crispy.

Super Crunchy Flounder Fillets

Servings:2
Cooking Time: 6 Minutes

Ingredients:
- ½ cup All-purpose flour or tapioca flour
- 1 Large egg white(s)
- 1 tablespoon Water
- ¾ teaspoon Table salt
- 1 cup Plain panko bread crumbs (gluten-free, if a concern)
- 2 4-ounce skinless flounder fillet(s)
- Vegetable oil spray

Directions:
1. Preheat the air fryer to 400°F.
2. Set up and fill three shallow soup plates or small pie plates on your counter: one for the flour; one for the egg white(s), beaten with the water and salt until foamy; and one for the bread crumbs.
3. Dip one fillet in the flour, turning it to coat both sides. Gently shake off any excess flour, then dip the fillet in the egg white mixture, turning it to coat. Let any excess egg white mixture slip back into the rest, then set the fish in the bread crumbs. Turn it several times, gently pressing it into the crumbs to create an even crust. Generously coat both sides of the fillet with vegetable oil spray. If necessary, set it aside and continue coating the remaining fillet(s) in the same way.
4. Set the fillet(s) in the basket. If working with more than one fillet, they should not touch, although they may be quite close together, depending on the basket's size. Air-fry undisturbed for 6 minutes, or until lightly browned and crunchy.
5. Use a nonstick-safe spatula to transfer the fillet(s) to a wire rack. Cool for only a minute or two before serving.

Quick Shrimp Scampi

Servings: 2
Cooking Time: 5 Minutes

Ingredients:
- 16 to 20 raw large shrimp, peeled, deveined and tails removed
- ½ cup white wine
- freshly ground black pepper
- ¼ cup + 1 tablespoon butter, divided
- 1 clove garlic, sliced
- 1 teaspoon olive oil
- salt, to taste
- juice of ½ lemon, to taste
- ¼ cup chopped fresh parsley

Directions:
1. Start by marinating the shrimp in the white wine and freshly ground black pepper for at least 30 minutes, or as long as 2 hours in the refrigerator.
2. Preheat the air fryer to 400°F.
3. Melt ¼ cup of butter in a small saucepan on the stovetop. Add the garlic and let the butter simmer, but be sure to not let it burn.
4. Pour the shrimp and marinade into the air fryer, letting the marinade drain through to the bottom drawer. Drizzle the olive oil on the shrimp and season well with salt. Air-fry at 400°F for 3 minutes. Turn the shrimp over (don't shake the basket because the marinade will splash around) and pour the garlic butter over the shrimp. Air-fry for another 2 minutes.
5. Remove the shrimp from the air fryer basket and transfer them to a bowl. Squeeze lemon juice over all the shrimp and toss with the chopped parsley and remaining tablespoon of butter. Season to taste with salt and serve immediately.

Beer-breaded Halibut Fish Tacos

Servings: 4

Cooking Time: 10 Minutes

Ingredients:

- 1 pound halibut, cut into 1-inch strips
- 1 cup light beer
- 1 jalapeño, minced and divided
- 1 clove garlic, minced
- ¼ teaspoon ground cumin
- ½ cup cornmeal
- ¼ cup all-purpose flour
- 1¼ teaspoons sea salt, divided
- 2 cups shredded cabbage
- 1 lime, juiced and divided
- ¼ cup Greek yogurt
- ¼ cup mayonnaise
- 1 cup grape tomatoes, quartered
- ½ cup chopped cilantro
- ¼ cup chopped onion
- 1 egg, whisked
- 8 corn tortillas

Directions:

1. In a shallow baking dish, place the fish, the beer, 1 teaspoon of the minced jalapeño, the garlic, and the cumin. Cover and refrigerate for 30 minutes.

2. Meanwhile, in a medium bowl, mix together the cornmeal, flour, and ½ teaspoon of the salt.

3. In large bowl, mix together the shredded cabbage, 1 tablespoon of the lime juice, the Greek yogurt, the mayonnaise, and ½ teaspoon of the salt.

4. In a small bowl, make the pico de gallo by mixing together the tomatoes, cilantro, onion, ¼ teaspoon of the salt, the remaining jalapeño, and the remaining lime juice.

5. Remove the fish from the refrigerator and discard the marinade. Dredge the fish in the whisked egg; then dredge the fish in the cornmeal flour mixture, until all pieces of fish have been breaded.

6. Preheat the air fryer to 350°F.

7. Place the fish in the air fryer basket and spray liberally with cooking spray. Cook for 6 minutes, flip and shake the fish, and cook another 4 minutes.

8. While the fish is cooking, heat the tortillas in a heavy skillet for 1 to 2 minutes over high heat.

9. To assemble the tacos, place the battered fish on the heated tortillas, and top with slaw and pico de gallo. Serve immediately.

Bacon-wrapped Scallops

Servings: 4

Cooking Time: 8 Minutes

Ingredients:

- 16 large scallops
- 8 bacon strips
- ½ teaspoon black pepper
- ¼ teaspoon smoked paprika

Directions:

1. Pat the scallops dry with a paper towel. Slice each of the bacon strips in half. Wrap 1 bacon strip around 1 scallop and secure with a toothpick. Repeat with the remaining scallops. Season the scallops with pepper and paprika.

2. Preheat the air fryer to 350°F.

3. Place the bacon-wrapped scallops in the air fryer basket and cook for 4 minutes, shake the basket, cook another 3 minutes, shake the basket, and cook another 1 to 3 to minutes. When the bacon is crispy, the scallops should be cooked through and slightly firm, but not rubbery. Serve immediately.

Maple-crusted Salmon

Servings: 2
Cooking Time: 8 Minutes
Ingredients:
- 12 ounces salmon filets
- ⅓ cup maple syrup
- 1 teaspoon Worcestershire sauce
- 2 teaspoons Dijon mustard or brown mustard
- ½ cup finely chopped walnuts
- ½ teaspoon sea salt
- ½ lemon
- 1 tablespoon chopped parsley, for garnish

Directions:
1. Place the salmon in a shallow baking dish. Top with maple syrup, Worcestershire sauce, and mustard. Refrigerate for 30 minutes.
2. Preheat the air fryer to 350°F.
3. Remove the salmon from the marinade and discard the marinade.
4. Place the chopped nuts on top of the salmon filets, and sprinkle salt on top of the nuts. Place the salmon, skin side down, in the air fryer basket. Cook for 6 to 8 minutes or until the fish flakes in the center.
5. Remove the salmon and plate on a serving platter. Squeeze fresh lemon over the top of the salmon and top with chopped parsley. Serve immediately.

Tilapia Teriyaki

Servings: 3
Cooking Time: 10 Minutes
Ingredients:
- 4 tablespoons teriyaki sauce
- 1 tablespoon pineapple juice
- 1 pound tilapia fillets
- cooking spray
- 6 ounces frozen mixed peppers with onions, thawed and drained
- 2 cups cooked rice

Directions:
1. Mix the teriyaki sauce and pineapple juice together in a small bowl.
2. Split tilapia fillets down the center lengthwise.
3. Brush all sides of fish with the sauce, spray air fryer basket with nonstick cooking spray, and place fish in the basket.
4. Stir the peppers and onions into the remaining sauce and spoon over the fish. Save any leftover sauce for drizzling over the fish when serving.
5. Cook at 360°F for 10 minutes, until fish flakes easily with a fork and is done in center.
6. Divide into 3 or 4 servings and serve each with approximately ½ cup cooked rice.

Honey Pecan Shrimp

Servings: 4
Cooking Time: 10 Minutes
Ingredients:
- ¼ cup cornstarch
- ¾ teaspoon sea salt, divided
- ¼ teaspoon pepper
- 2 egg whites
- ⅔ cup finely chopped pecans
- 1 pound raw, peeled, and deveined shrimp
- ¼ cup honey
- 2 tablespoons mayonnaise

Directions:
1. In a small bowl, whisk together the cornstarch, ½ teaspoon of the salt, and the pepper.
2. In a second bowl, whisk together the egg whites until soft and foamy. (They don't need to be whipped to peaks or even soft peaks, just frothy.)
3. In a third bowl, mix together the pecans and the remaining ¼ teaspoon of sea salt.
4. Pat the shrimp dry with paper towels. Working in small batches, dip the shrimp into

the cornstarch, then into the egg whites, and then into the pecans until all the shrimp are coated with pecans.

5. Preheat the air fryer to 330°F.

6. Place the coated shrimp inside the air fryer basket and spray with cooking spray. Cook for 5 minutes, toss the shrimp, and cook another 5 minutes.

7. Meanwhile, place the honey in a microwave-safe bowl and microwave for 30 seconds. Whisk in the mayonnaise until smooth and creamy. Pour the honey sauce into a serving bowl. Add the cooked shrimp to the serving bowl while hot and toss to coat. Serve immediately.

Fish Sticks For Grown-ups

Servings: 4

Cooking Time: 6 Minutes

Ingredients:

- 1 pound fish fillets
- ½ teaspoon hot sauce
- 1 tablespoon coarse brown mustard
- 1 teaspoon Worcestershire sauce
- salt
- Crumb Coating
- ¾ cup panko breadcrumbs
- ¼ cup stone-ground cornmeal
- ¼ teaspoon salt
- oil for misting or cooking spray

Directions:

1. Cut fish fillets crosswise into slices 1-inch wide.

2. Mix the hot sauce, mustard, and Worcestershire sauce together to make a paste and rub on all sides of the fish. Season to taste with salt.

3. Mix crumb coating ingredients together and spread on a sheet of wax paper.

4. Roll the fish fillets in the crumb mixture.

5. Spray all sides with olive oil or cooking spray and place in air fryer basket in a single layer.

6. Cook at 390°F for 6 minutes, until fish flakes easily.

Maple Balsamic Glazed Salmon

Servings: 4

Cooking Time: 10 Minutes

Ingredients:

- 4 (6-ounce) fillets of salmon
- salt and freshly ground black pepper
- vegetable oil
- ¼ cup pure maple syrup
- 3 tablespoons balsamic vinegar
- 1 teaspoon Dijon mustard

Directions:

1. Preheat the air fryer to 400°F.

2. Season the salmon well with salt and freshly ground black pepper. Spray or brush the bottom of the air fryer basket with vegetable oil and place the salmon fillets inside. Air-fry the salmon for 5 minutes.

3. While the salmon is air-frying, combine the maple syrup, balsamic vinegar and Dijon mustard in a small saucepan over medium heat and stir to blend well. Let the mixture simmer while the fish is cooking. It should start to thicken slightly, but keep your eye on it so it doesn't burn.

4. Brush the glaze on the salmon fillets and air-fry for an additional 5 minutes. The salmon should feel firm to the touch when finished and the glaze should be nicely browned on top. Brush a little more glaze on top before removing and serving with rice and vegetables, or a nice green salad.

Recipe Index

Printed by Libri Plureos GmbH in Hamburg,
Germany